PSYCHOLOGY FOR
THE PARAMEDICAL
PROFESSIONS

K.T. STRONGMAN

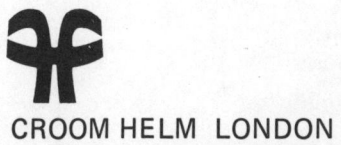

CROOM HELM LONDON

© 1979 K.T. Strongman
Croom Helm Ltd, 2-10 St John's Road, London SW11

British Library Cataloguing in Publication Data

Strongman, Kenneth Thomas
    Psychology for the paramedical professions.
    1. Psychology
    I. Title
    150'.2'461   BF131

    ISBN 0-85664-652-0

    ISBN 0-85664-852-3 Pbk

Printed and bound in Great Britain

CONTENTS

Preface

1. Psychology and Its Methods   9
2. Learning – Classical and Instrumental Conditioning   24
3. Behaviour Modification   45
4. The Management of Learning   64
5. Memory and Forgetting   76
6. Perception   94
7. Thinking   112
8. Emotion   130
9. Motivation   152
10. Personality Theory   166
11. Intelligence   182
12. Interpersonal Relationships   195
13. Judgements and Impressions of Personality   213
14. Learning and Training Social Skills   230
15. Attitudes and Prejudice   246
16. Leadership and Groups   262

References   279

Index   285

For Katherine Ingamells
and her Colleagues

PREFACE

The impetus for this book came from many years of helping in the teaching of psychology at St Loyes School of Occupational Therapy, plus occasional lectures to other members and trainee members of the paramedical professions. On many of these occasions I felt the need of a single text to which I might refer anyone who was interested. Of course, there is a plenitude of texts on introductory psychology, but very few of these are slanted specifically towards the paramedical services. The present aim is to provide such a book.

In attempting to realise this aim, I became aware of at least one of the reasons why few such books exist. There is only a very scanty body of psychological knowledge which has been drawn specifically from the medical world and its various supporting professions. Consequently, I have tried to direct this book at its intended audience in three ways: (a) by choosing topics which are most germane to their interests, (b) by choosing illustrative examples, wherever possible, from everyday life, or from hospital or related settings, and (c) by making particular provision in the study questions which appear at the end of each chapter.

My hope is that the contents of this book will simultaneously provide a reasonably thorough grounding in basic psychological research and ideas, and stimulate at least some students to read more and to pursue the subject of psychology in more depth.

1 PSYCHOLOGY AND ITS METHODS

Psychology is the (scientific) study of behaviour.

This initial chapter will be spent expanding, justifying and exploring the implications of this definition.

Behaviour

To begin at the end, the final word in the definition is 'behaviour'. This means that psychology as it is now pursued as an academic and applied discipline is *not* concerned with mind, soul, spirit, mental life or any other essentially philosophical concept. Wherever possible it is concerned with behaviour, since in human functioning it is behaviour that is tangible, observable and measurable. Psychologists constantly make reference to what can be seen and measured, and with minor exceptions they are similar in this to any other scientist, from biochemist to geologist. Also, it is not that psychologists would want to deny that people have minds, souls, spirits or what have you, but would want to suggest that such entities do not form the proper subject matter for psychological enquiry. They are the domain of the philosopher or theologist; they are intangibles.

Perhaps what has been said so far may give the impression that psychology is very dry. It is not; at least it is no drier than any other academic or scientific discipline, and in the opinion of many, considerably more interesting. Certainly psychologists are mainly concerned with the palpable aspects of human functioning, but of course they cannot always go as far in this direction as they would wish.

Take for example two processes which are very much a part of human psychology: learning and memory. Although in studying these, psychologists are much concerned to find ways in which they can be cunningly reflected in behaviour, whatever techniques of study they devise, they can only ever look at such processes indirectly. Quite accurately, I referred to learning and memory as *processes*. Processes cannot be observed directly, they can only be *inferred* from direct observations of behaviour. As will become clear, inference is a very important topic in psychology. It is not that the psychologist believes that there is nothing more to man than his behaviour, but rather that he feels that for the most part, he can only gain an understanding of man by observing his behaviour. What else is there?

Having said that psychology is mainly concerned with behaviour may seem to have imposed a massive limitation on the subject. That this is not so is attested to by the presence of this book and many others like it. In broad terms the psychologist is interested in all man's basic processes: learning, perception, motivation, emotion, intellectual or cognitive abilities, memory, language and personality. He is interested, not only in these processes in a static sense, but also in their development. And he is concerned with the abnormalities that might result when they go wrong in some way. And finally he is interested in the processes that come into play when one person interacts with another, i.e. in social behaviour.

Overall, the psychologist is concerned with any activities of, or responses made by, organisms, usually, but not always, human organisms, that can be seen by observers or measured with whatever instruments the psychologists can reasonably devise.

(Scientific) Study

Having established what psychologists are concerned with, it is important to say something of the way in which they express their concern. If you think of any other science, particularly a natural or biological science rather than a social science, it is very clear that it is concerned primarily with laboratory experimentation, often involving extremely complex measuring instruments. Psychology is often like this as well, but for two reasons it is also a little different. First, it is a relatively young discipline, perhaps 100 years old as a science, and therefore has not reached the same sophistication of knowledge and method as have disciplines such as physics or biology. However, it *has* been in the fortunate position of being able to learn from these other subjects. Second, the subject matter of psychology is man, the most unusual, idiosyncratic and complex creature on earth. Not surprisingly therefore there are ways of studying man that a physicist could not use in studying a gas or a geologist could not use in studying a rock.

Observation

The starting-point for any psychological enquiry, when it has gone beyond being an idea in a psychologist's head, is observation. The psychologist has to go and actually observe what a person or a group of people are doing. However intricate his measurements and analysis eventually become, he must start by observing. Indeed because of the complexities of what is involved some investigations in psychology never get beyond the observational level.

It may sound easy enough to observe — you just look at a bit of behaviour. Unfortunately however, it is rather more complex than that. Since the essence of science is to be systematic so that others can know *exactly* what you have done in order to repeat it for themselves if they wish, great care has to be taken in exactly *what* is observed and *how* it is observed.

For example, suppose that you were interested in a very small response such as the rate at which a person blinked under various conditions. You might want to compare this when the person was reading and when in conversation. This is reasonable enough but you would have to begin by being very clear what you meant by reading and under what conditions, and similarly with conversation. Not too difficult. However, and more important, you would have to decide exactly what a blink was. This may sound laughable – a blink is a blink is a blink. Not so; if you look at a few blinks you will see what the problem is. Do the eyes have to be completely closed or not? How far? How fast does the blink have to be? Does one count eye twitches and eye rubbing and langorous blinks that seem to be done for social effect?

It is not only a matter of defining the behaviour, it is a question of deciding precisely when it should be observed. Do you make your observations for an hour, continuously, or for an hour at five or ten minute intervals? At what time of day? What do you do about any blinks that you might have missed when you yourself were blinking or sneezing or somesuch? And so on. Yet this is one of the simplest responses one can think of; just blinking. Nevertheless, all these questions have to be dealt with if any sort of accuracy and precision is to be achieved. You might ask why it is necessary to be as accurate as all that; would not a rough guide do as well? The answer, of course, is that it would not. One wants to be able to make firm and meaningful generalisations about what people do, and for these generalisations to be of some use. In which case they have to be as precise as they can be. If a physicist or a chemist were sloppy or haphazard in his observations, the world might eventually be destroyed. A sloppy psychologist could have an even more hazardous effect.

Consider a rather more complex example. Imagine that a psychologist became interested in the frequency of children's aggression in the school playground. He would have a very similar set of problems to deal with as those he would have if studying blinking, but they would be even more difficult. He would have to begin by defining aggression, which as will be seen in a later chapter, is no easy matter. Then he would have to set up some exact categories of what he meant by the behaviour. What *exactly* is an aggressive blow? How does one measure and observe verbal aggression? What distinguishes it from other verbal behaviour? When should the observations be made, and how often and at what type of school, and so on?

In the case of eye-blinks or playground aggression, it does not really matter how the psychologist sorts out these problems, as long as it is done with common sense. What does matter is that once he has made his various decisions he records them accurately and then sticks to them; in other words, that he is consistent. Then anyone else can follow on and repeat what he has done, however arbitrary the initial decisions might have been. Another crucial aspect of science is that it is *repeatable*.

As stated above, the starting-point for any psychological investigation is observation. Thereafter the investigation can take a number of different directions. It may for example stay at the level of *naturalistic* observation (aggression in the playground) simply because it is impossible to proceed in any other way. If one is interested in the psychological effects of the introduction of television into a rural area there would never be the time and money to set up a rural area and study it with and without television. It has to be studied naturally; a procedure which is relatively lacking in precision.

Psychological research may take the form of *case histories* with interest centred on a global sort of approach to one individual rather than on an analysis of him into his separate faculties. This of course might be open to all manner of biases, from a person's mistaken memories, to his desire to say the 'right' thing or to present himself or his family in a particular light. Sometimes such an approach is the only one open, but it is necessarily subjective rather than objective. And to be *objective* is another great tenet of scientific method.

Typically the psychologist's own are various test methods aimed at measuring the individual's abilities, interests, attitudes and accomplishments in comparison with those of other individuals. The aim here is to tap a sample of the individual's behaviour, or at least his answers to questions about his behaviour, in order to predict from this what he might or might not do, given the opportunity. Psychological tests are a very important part of the subject and will be returned to at several places in this book.

Experimentation

From the viewpoint of conventional scientific method there is one thing wrong with observation, and with the other techniques mentioned above; although made as precise as possible, they lack the precision which can be achieved within a laboratory. In his laboratory the psychologist can exercise a far more effective control over the environment and the conditions in which he is interested, than he can when he is out in the real world. Thus it is often the aim of psychological investigations to reach that stage in which actual laboratory experiments can be run.

Before going on to describe the usual form of psychological experiments it must be pointed out that they involve one basic difficulty. By their very nature they are artificial. As soon as a person (at this stage he would be called a subject) is persuaded to enter a psychological laboratory to take part in an experiment, he is in an artificial situation. On the one hand, the laboratory enables far more exact measures to be taken than are possible in real life and so any generalisations that are made or conclusions that are drawn have more substance. On the other hand, these conclusions are of questionable applicability to real life. Are the behaviours which have been observed in the laboratory necessarily as they would have been in real life? Is it meaningful to abstract from the one situation to the other? The psychologist always faces this problem of the relative advantages and disadvantages of carrying out his investigations in the laboratory or in the real world.

Any experiment in psychology, or indeed in any other discipline, has three essential parts. It is important to understand these from the start.
(1) The *independent* variable – that which the experimenter manipulates.
(2) The *dependent* variable – that which the experimenter measures.
(3) *Control* conditions – conditions which the experimenter imposes so that he can be sure that whatever results he obtains are due solely to the manipulations he has carried out.

These three aspects of experimentation will become clear with an example.

Think of the very practical question: does learning to play badminton interfere with a person's capacity at tennis? At first sight it might seem that one could answer this question by persuading someone to learn badminton up to some recognised level of performance and then see how he got on when he attempted to play tennis. Recognising that there might be male/female and age differences, one might even persuade a group of varied persons to undergo this procedure. However, for a number of reasons it would be impossible to draw any conclusions from such an investigation.

For example, how would one know that the badminton had *interfered* (enhancing or impeding) the tennis? How would one know that the subjects might not have learned tennis with exactly the same facility (or lack of it) *without* the previous experience of learning badminton? Do people improve at a sport simply with the passage of time? Or do they deteriorate? And so on.

In fact there is a standard experimental design which allows a problem such as this to be investigated in such a way that it is possible to draw proper conclusions from it. Hence:

Experimental group: Learns tennis.   Learns badminton.   Tested on tennis.

This is quite straightforward. A group of subjects is asked to learn to play tennis up to a given criterion of performance. Then they learn to play badminton up to a given criterion, following which they are tested on tennis.

Control group: Learns tennis.   Rests.   Tested on tennis.

The control group, consisting of the same number and type of people as the experimental group (chosen either at random from the general population or because of some special quality, such as never having played racket sports previously) learn to play tennis to the same criterion as used in the experimental group. They then rest (that is, play no racket sports) for the same amount of time that it takes the experimental group to learn to play badminton. And finally they are tested on tennis as are the experimental group.

In this simple experiment the *independent variable* is the order in which the groups learn tennis and badminton or learn tennis and do nothing. The *dependent variable* is whatever measure the experimenter takes of their tennis ability when he tests them. The *control* procedure is obvious, depending in this case on the use of a group equivalent to the experimental group. This is controlling for the simple passage of time (and anything which it might by chance contain) between the initial learning and the final testing.

Now, if at the time of test the experimental group scores better than the control group it would be legitimate to conclude that the badminton has facilitated their tennis (the control group has no badminton). On the other hand, if they do worse on test than the control group, then it is legitimate to conclude that the badminton has impeded their tennis. Either way, this provides some initial data on the possibility of transfer of skills between one racket sport and another.

Whatever specific form it takes any experiment in psychology has these same basic elements. Experimentation such as this, although seeming to allow valid conclusions to be drawn has two major problems associated with it. These are problems which apply to any research in psychology.

First there is the question of *measurement.* Any science is only as good as its measuring instruments, and psychology is no exception to this. The aim is therefore continuously to modify and refine any measures of man's abilities that are developed. However, it is a simpler matter to make measurements of physical qualities such as weight or height than it is to measure psychological capacities. How, for example, can one measure learning or memory or the strength of a person's motivation? At best one can only measure these aspects of human functioning indirectly. Much of psychology then is taken up with cunning schemes to devise better and more subtle measures of the processes which might be of interest. As might be imagined with a source of data as complex as a human being, this aim is often difficult to realise.

As a further example, just take the hypothetical experiment described above. How does one measure ability at tennis? There are many ways. For example: points gained from a known player; errors made in the course of an hour; accuracy of ball placement; success in open competitition; and so on. Choices have to be made.

Second, in the description above, it was said 'if the experimental group does *better* than the control group' or 'does *worse*'. What *exactly* is meant by better or worse in the context of a psychological experiment? Is 50 per cent better, acceptably better, or would only 10 per cent do? Fortunately psychologists have a way of making decisions such as these; that is, by the use of *statistics.*

At the everyday level, if people consider statistics at all, they tend to think of *descriptive statistics.* These are figures that describe, for example, how many people on average smoke cigarettes, or how many people in England die from bronchitis in comparison with France. Of course, there is an important place in psychology for such descriptive statistics. However, of equal importance are what are known as *inferential statistics.* These are techniques which have been devised by statisticians and psychologists (in some cases) which allow them to say how much better is better or how much worse is worse. It enables them to say whether or not they can draw valid conclusions from their data; to say in fact whether their experimental manipulation was a significant one or whether their findings might just have come about by chance in spite of what they did.

Both descriptive and inferential statistics have an important role to play in psychological research. Any generalisation which a psychologist makes is very different from those that might be made in everyday life. They are more precise, are based on more systematic observations, and limits can be placed on the extent to which they can be regarded as valid. Although any psychological research starts with everyday observation, to take its proper place within what might be termed a body of psychological knowledge, it has to move some distance from everyday life.

Models of Man

In a discipline with a subject matter as complex as that of psychology there are inevitably many difficulties and problems. Some of these will be discussed as this book progresses. However, there is one overriding problem which should be considered before all else. This concerns the various models of man that psychologists can adopt.

The best way into the problem is to think for a moment of the *aims* of psychology. From what has been said so far about the methods psychologists use, the aims of the subject, insofar as it is regarded as a science, are those of any science: *observation* in order to make *predictions* in order ultimately to *exercise control*. People are observed in what they do, theories are constructed and hypotheses tested, in order to be able to make predictions about what people will do in the future. The goal of such prediction is not just *understanding* and knowledge, but also control. If it is known what aspects of an individual's experiences and make-up lead to schizophrenia or neurosis, or educational retardation, or a lack of social skill, then something can perhaps be done to change the person, to make him happier and more socially acceptable.

Determinism Versus Free-will

The fundamental problem is that of whether or not it *is* possible to make more and more precise predictions about human functioning. If one believes that this is possible then one is basically avowing what would be termed a deterministic belief. That is, one is *assuming* that man has no free will, that his basic actions are determined. This does not mean that in any sense they are pre-ordained (by a deity for example) but rather that, given certain conditions, then a person has no choice in what he does. Although he seems to make a choice at all manner of points in his life, an outsider who knew him well enough could predict what he would choose.

Of course the main question then becomes, what does 'know him

well enough' mean? It means to those who make the deterministic
assumption that a person's actions are the result of (1) his genetic make-
up (whatever propensities he inherits), (2) his past experiences, and (3)
his present environment and general situation, all of which interact to
make him do whatever he does.

There are three major difficulties with this argument. First, it is
based on the *assumption* of determinism, and this may be unwarranted.
It may be that, as some people believe, including some psychologists,
man does have an element of free will in his make-up.

Second, even if it is accepted that man is basically predictable then
will it ever be possible to predict what he does with any degree of
accuracy *in the individual case*? As has already been shown, psychologists are mainly concerned with predicting what groups of people will
do on average and setting statistical limits on their predictions. The
ultimate aim though would be that of individual prediction. At the outset it should be said that man is probably too complex for this aim ever
to be achieved. If one were to build a computer which contained *everything* there were to know of a single person, one would have virtually
built the person himself. This would seem unlikely, although not necessarily impossible.

Finally, there is the question of control. If one of the aims of prediction is control then there are immediate ethical problems. Who controls whom, and to what end? Of course, considerations such as this
involve serious moral judgements about which there is little point in
rehearsing the arguments here. However, they are important issues
about which each individual has to make up his mind; this includes
psychologists.

Behaviourism

The deterministic model of man reached its extreme position with the
advent in the 1920s of behaviourism, a movement which has had an
extremely important influence on psychology. This influence was felt
(and still is) not just as a reaction to the rather woolly suppositions of
Freudian psychoanalysis, but because of its emphasis on scientific
method. The tenets of behaviourism can be fairly easily itemised.
(1) Man *is* his *behaviour.* This means that it is possible to learn all that
there is to know of someone through a study of his behaviour. This
viewpoint can be expressed so:

S-----------R

Any stimulus from the environment (which of course is observable) brings about a response in the organism (which of course is observable). If, by observation, the psychologists can establish the precise relationships which exist between stimuli and responses then they will know all there is to know about human functioning. Clearly this is a very mechanistic model of man, viewing him very much as a machine which has inputs and outputs, and even suggesting that to find out the relationship between input and output, it is unnecessary to know much about how the machine is constructed.

This viewpoint has pushed psychology in the direction of increasing rigour in its research methods. Indeed, to some extent most twentieth-century psychologists could be fairly described as *methodological* behaviourists. Some though go further, accepting all the tenets about man which it is possible to hold from the behaviourist viewpoint. These are *radical* behaviourists.

(2) Man is *predictable*. This point has already been made. The belief is that it is possible to predict man at least on the level of good statistical prediction, but ultimately on the level of precise individual prediction.

(3) Man lives in an *objective* world. That is, man lives in a reliable, tangible world of observations, facts and data in which measurement is possible and in which one man can gain knowledge of another man.

(4) Man is *rational*. That is, man acts according to laws of reason, intelligence and logic. He acts on his empirical knowledge of the world and does not simply behave at random, or capriciously.

(5) Men are *alike*. Although in detail each man is unique, he is sufficiently similar to other men that it is possible through observation to find laws governing what he does and to make valid generalisations about him.

(6) Man can be *analysed* into distinct characteristics. This means that man has a definite number of capacities which can be investigated separately. Doing this will lose no information about the individual.

(7) Man is an *evolved* creature and should be studied as such.

(8) Man is *knowable scientifically*.

Phenomenological Psychology

In recent years there has sprung up a reaction against behaviourism. This has taken many guises but these can be broadly drawn together under the umbrella term of phenomenology. This represents viewpoints in which stress is placed on man's *experiences* rather than his behaviour. The major implication is that each of us *perceives* the world in a unique way, although our perceptions might have points in common. And it is these perceptions, or the *intentions* to which they give rise that determine how we react and what we are.

This can be expressed: S----------O----------R

A stimulus impinges on the organism which perceives it, processes it, decides what to do about it, and then attempts to fulfil its intention. The *O* is an important intervening point between stimulus and response; it is where choices are made.

Before going on to itemise the basic assumptions of this alternative model of man, an example may help to highlight the essential differences between the behaviourist and the phenomenological psychologist. Imagine that a psychologist wishes to carry out some preliminary observations on the effects of anger on intellectual performance. As a task he chooses making a precis of some complex passage of prose. His subjects are five students chosen because they are in the same study group. They are male, aged 20 and of similar backgrounds. Half-way through their precis he makes them angry by arranging to have one of their peers stop them, read through what they have so far produced and be sarcastic about it. He also has a matched control group, interrupted at the same point by the same person but without the sarcasm.

From the viewpoint of conventional science and behaviourism this is a perfectly reasonable preliminary investigation which could be developed into a complete research programme. However, from the viewpoint of the experiential psychologist a great deal is missing. For example, the experimental group might contain two or three men who see themselves as shaky students, surprised to have come so far. They expect to do badly on intellectual tasks. So, they are not surprised to be castigated, even by one of their peers. Sarcasm has no effect on them; they have come to expect it.

On the other hand, the control group might contain a man or two who believed themselves to be worthwile, perceptive, intelligent students; a cut above the general run. They will resent and be made angry by *any* interruption from a peer, sarcastic or otherwise, and their precis-making will suffer accordingly. Or any of the subjects might be the sort of people who have an overwhelming respect for authority. So they are made a little anxious simply by being asked to take part in an experiment. Their intellectual performance is worse than it would normally be, whatever is done to them.

It could be said that all of these possibilities are merely elements in the situation which the investigator has not thought to control and which he might have to at some time. From the viewpoint of the phenomenological psychologist, each of these elements is perceptual or experiential. Each of the subjects has his background of unique experiences which are causing him to view the situation in a unique way. His perceptions are determining his individual reactions. So, a person of this persuasion would argue that psychologists should attempt to see the world through the other person's eyes.

Again, the main tenets of phenomenological psychology can be easily summarised. It is important to compare these with the main tenets of behaviourism a few pages back.

(1) Man is his *consciousness.* Consciousness is defined in this context as a feeling of being active, an awareness of one's identity and the understanding which this gives.

(2) Man is *unpredictable.* Man has choice, free will and makes active decisions. It should be remembered that this is just as much of an assumption as the alternative, that man *is* predictable. It does lead to some interesting considerations. For example, does the knowledge by a man that his behaviour is in some way predictable, lead him to change the behaviour? If so, in what direction? Or would knowledge of this knowledge allow his behaviour once again to be predictable?

Related to this, it is assumed that man's acts are *intentional.* That is, he assesses a situation, arrives at a decision and then does whatever he intends to do, unless of course something happens to stop him.

(3) Man lives in a *subjective* world. The important aspects of the world are private experiences, emotions, feelings and perceptions. So the proper study of psychologists is experience and perception. The important question, of course, is *how* is this achieved?

(4) Man is *arational.* He contradicts the laws of reason in what he does. He has faith, religions, beliefs, and makes value judgements, all of which it is important to study.

(5) Man is *unique,* and should be studied as such.

(6) Man should be studied as a *whole*. If man is broken down into his parts and these parts are studied separately, something is lost from the true picture of man. The whole is greater than the sum of the parts in this case.

(7) Man is still *evolving*, still engaged in becoming something different and should be studied as such.

(8) Man is *more* than can ever be known by man, a limitation which should be realised from the start.

Behaviourism and the experiential or phenomenological approach represent two completely opposed viewpoints in psychology, or more properly, two completely opposite models of man. One has led to the rules and methods of conventional science being applied to the study of man. The other has sprung up partly as a reaction to this, and seeks to put 'man' back into the picture and leave out the machine.

Since each of these models rests on assumptions, and assumptions are beliefs, then there is no right or wrong about them. One simply has to make a decision about which is the more appropriate, for whatever reason. Or to make no decisions at all and reach a compromise position. There would be no harm in this since either approach generates more information about human psychology. It must be said however, that the deterministic approach has generated far more than the experiential, and no doubt will continue to do so. Even if it is appropriate to make the attempt it is very difficult to see the world through another person's eyes.

Perhaps the most fundamental difference between these two models is to be seen in some of their implications. On the face of it, the deterministic, behaviouristic approach is much tougher than the experiential. It suggests rigorous scientific enquiry. And yet it implies that man cannot be *blamed* for his actions. If he has no free will then it makes no sense to blame him for whatever he does or to hold him *responsible*. Equally, of course, it makes no sense to admire him for his bravery. The brave man or the coward is only doing all that is open to him in the situation, given his make-up and previous experience. This means, amongst other things, that it would be wrong to hold criminals responsible for their actions (and not just those with 'diminished' responsibility.)

By contrast, the much softer-seeming phenomenological approach has very tough implications. Man can be held responsible for his actions, he has choice and free will. His bravery is therefore to be valued, and his cowardice to be decried. He can be held blameworthy and accountable.

As a final point on these two models of man, perhaps it should be said that most psychologists adhere to neither one nor the other as strongly as they have been described here. These are the extremes, and most psychologists advocate the use of scientifically based enquiry within psychology, even if sometimes they might believe that such enquiry should be adapted to study intentions of subjective experiences, as far as this might be possible.

Conclusions

The reasons why the definition of psychology given at the start of this chapter was written: 'the (scientific) study of behaviour' should by now be obvious. Although the status of modern psychology has been founded on a scientific study, there are some who believe that this is a limited approach and that man can never be fully knowable with science; it makes him too machine-like.

However, the aim of this book is to reflect the current state of psychological knowledge as it is thought to be relevant particularly to the paramedical services. Consequently, much of what follows is based upon investigations which have been made within the framework of conventional science. Very few investigations have been made outside this framework. The first chapters give a general picture of the various aspects of psychological functioning which tend to have been studied as reasonably discrete topics. And finally there are some five chapters which deal with man's social behaviour; his interaction with other men.

Summary Points

(1) Psychology is the (scientific) study of behaviour.
(2) By behaviour is meant what is observable and measurable, which ultimately is the psychologist's only way to get at any processes which might go on inside the individual.
(3) For the most part psychological research is based on systematic observation and controlled experimentation although it has some methods such as case studies and interviews which are its own.
(4) The three important aspects of an experiment are: independent variable, dependent variable, and control of unwanted variables.
(5) Many psychological generalisations are based on statistics which can be used to describe data or to make inferences about its significance.
(6) In current psychology there are two very different models of man which are based on quite different assumptions; the deterministic, best exemplified by behaviourism, and that which gives man free will, best exemplified by the experientialists or phenomenological psychologists.
(7) Although these two approaches exist and have quite different implications, the bulk of psychological knowledge has come from a framework of conventional science, even though many of those who have used this approach might have given little thought to whether or not man has free will.

Study Questions – 1

(1) What is psychology? What ways of studying human behaviour would be of most benefit to your profession?
(2) Choose some aspect of behaviour which is relatively common in a

hospital setting and carry out a *systematic* observation of it. Try to be thorough enough to make a meaningful generalisation.

(3) Design an experiment to assess the effects of hospitalisation on a person's intellectual capacities. What would you have to control for in such a study?

(4) Do you think that man's behaviour is determined, or that he has free will? If you believe that he is more than a machine, say what he has that a machine has not, and how it can be studied. Illustrate your answers by examples chosen from amongst hospital patients or staff.

(5) Do you think that psychologists' understanding and knowledge will ever be full enough such that the psychological impact of hospitalisation will be fully explored?

(6) In what ways might learning about psychology change your own individual psychology and the way in which you deal with your patients, colleagues and friends?

(7) What are the main ways in which psychology is relevant to your profession? Are there any ways in which it could help you in that profession?

(8) What do you think are psychology's main applications to society in general?

(9) Would you consider the prediction and control of a patient's behaviour to be an important and worthwhile endeavour?

(10) Do you think that hospitals in general, and your profession in particular would benefit from psychological research? If you do, give examples of what most needs to be done. If you do not, say why not and say how any remaining professional problems could best be answered.

2 LEARNING – CLASSICAL AND INSTRUMENTAL CONDITIONING

Learning is a process which is believed to determine any relatively permanent changes in behaviour which result from practice or experience. As ever, it is only what the organism does (its performance) that can be observed and measured so, like many other psychological processes, learning is inferred from behaviour. Because learning is such a universal phenomenon (it is probable that all animals and even some plants learn), it is always tempting to make broad generalisations about it. However, this must be done with caution, otherwise the concept would lose its meaning by becoming over inclusive.

Consider for a moment the definition given above. The key phrase is 'permanent changes in behaviour'. The words 'permanent change' are important because there are many changes which occur in behaviour which are *transient* or temporary, having nothing to do with learning and which should not be confused with it. Think for example of the alterations in behaviour due to fatigue, or too much alcohol, or to worry about examinations. After rest, the passage of time and the taking of the examinations, behaviour reverts to normal – no learning has taken place.

As well as fairly obvious points such as the one just made, there are other changes in performance in which it is difficult to see whether or not learning has taken place or is even involved. Take the example of a person learning a new sport. Clearly, much of the initial improvement in his game can reasonably be attributed to learning. But once he has reached a fair proficiency his performance still fluctuates. Learning might also be involved in these later changes, but so also might be motivation, physiological state, the incentive involved in a particular match, where it is being played, and so on. Each of these factors would have to be taken into account before conclusions could be drawn about the learning process. And related to such variables are the even more important ones of *growth* and *maturation*. When a child has learned something new, over time he may show a steady improvement at it, but simply because he is growing and maturing physically. It is important to separate the effects of maturation from those of learning.

In everyday language, learning is often defined as profiting by experience. Although at first sight this definition might seem adequate, its glibness is only confusing. It is difficult to determine what, in this context, is meant by 'profit', and in fact, however the word is defined it is clear that much learning does *not* profit the learner. Some people learn to bite their nails for example, or learn social habits that lead others to dislike them. Some psychologists would even go so far as to say that conditions like neurosis, psychosis, alcoholism and obesity are learned; it is obvious that little profit is to be found in these.

For the most part, psychologists today emphasise interpretations of learning as *habit formation* – that is, the acquiring of a connection between stimuli and responses, a connection which did not previously exist for the individual. The simplest example of this is perhaps that of the child learning to refer to objects in the environment in the correct way, according to the language of his culture. He learns for example that certain objects made of wood and graphite (the stimuli) are usually referred to as pencils (the response). Apart from the learning of complex responses and skills (which are dealt with in Chapter 4), there are two main types of such learning. These are termed classical and instrumental conditioning and will be described in turn, even though, in real life they will both usually be involved in any one simple bit of learning.

Classical Conditioning

The Basic Process

Classical conditioning is also known as *Pavlovian* conditioning, after Pavlov who was its progenitor, and *respondent* conditioning because of its concern with responses which are elicited from the organism by stimuli. It is the most simple, basic and straightforward sort of learning involving little more than association and simple reflexes.

At about the turn of the century, Pavlov, who was primarily a physiologist, noticed that hungry dogs would salivate not only when food was placed into their mouths, but also when they could merely see the food. He thought that this must be a learned response and would be worthy of study.

Pavlov constructed a harness into which dogs could be strapped, placed this in a sound-proof room, and exposed the salivary glands of the dogs to the surface of their cheeks so that measurement of salivary secretion could be made easily. Then, typically, Pavlov would turn on a light (which could be seen by the food-deprived dog), and follow this almost immediately with an automatic delivery of some meat powder into the dog's mouth. The dog would eat. Pavlov termed the light a conditioning stimulus (CS) and the meat powder an unconditioned stimulus (US).

To begin with, on each such trial involving the pairing of the CS and US the dog would only salivate when the food was in its mouth. But after a number of trials it would begin to salivate at the sight of the light and *before* it had received the food. This, Pavlov termed a conditioned response (CR), salivation following the US being called an unconditioned response (UR).

This then is the basic procedure for establishing a classically conditioned response, a procedure which has been employed successfully hundreds and thousands of times in the laboratory on a variety of responses (from eye-blinks, to knee-jerks, to vomiting) and of course even more often in the natural circumstances of everyday life. The procedure can be represented diagramatically as below, in which the example is of Pavlov's original study.

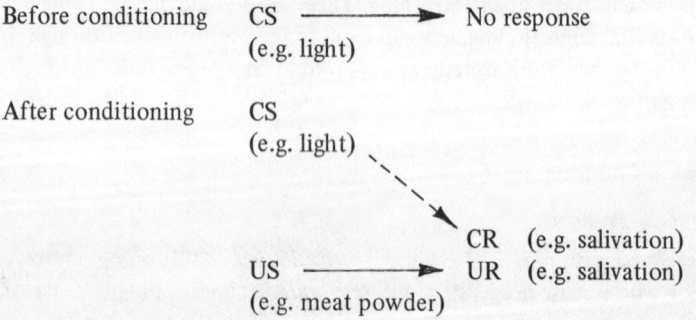

Notice that in classical conditioning the CS and the US are similar (both salivation in the original studies), although they are not precisely the same. The UR is stronger than the CR, that is, for example, more saliva is secreted. Also, notice that the learning comes about through an association of one stimulus (CS) with another, more powerful stimulus (US), which already evokes a response from the organism. This order of association is known as *reinforcement* in classical conditioning.

To define classical conditioning then, it is the build up of an association between a neutral stimulus (CS) and a response (CR) through a number of occasions on which the CS has been paired in a controlled manner with a stimulus (US) which already elicits the response in question. To give a real life example of this type of learning, imagine a person in hospital who has to have regular, painful injections. When the needle goes in (US) it elicits from him responses such as sweating, trembling, tensing muscles etc. (URs). After a few such experiences he will come to make similar responses (now CRs) at the sight of the nurse walking towards him with the hypodermic needle (CSs). Put less precisely, he has learned to fear the sight of a hypodermic needle. In fact, it is often with basic, relatively crude emotional responses that classical conditioning is concerned. Consider an even more common example; many people have painful experiences when they go to the dentist. It does not take many such experiences before they become anxious (CRs) at the distinctive smells of the surgery (CSs), and at the sight of the drill (CS), or even of the dentist himself (CS).

Phenomena of Classical Conditioning

(1) Measurement. In writings about classical conditioning it is often stated that any stimulus can be associated with any respondent but that to be optimally effective, the US should follow about half a second behind the CS. What exactly is meant by effective? Clearly, it refers to how well the response is learned, in other words how *strong* and how *frequent* are the CRs. If they occur infrequently and weakly then the learning has not been particularly effective.

There are four common measures of classical conditioning, some permutations of which are taken in most investigations.

(a) *Size* of the CR, this being the obvious measure of response strength. In Pavlov's original studies this was given simply by amount of saliva secreted. In other studies it is not so easy to assess, with a knee-jerk for example.

(b) *Latency* of CRs. This refers to the speed with which the CR follows the CS, a faster response (shorter latency) taken as indicative of greater strength.

(c) *Trials to a criterion.* A count is sometimes made of the number of trials (pairings between CS and US) needed before the first CR is made, fewer such trials indicating faster conditioning and greater response strength.

(d) *Probability of occurrence* of the CR. Often, in classical conditioning CRs are not made every time the CS appears, so it is possible to determine the proportion of trials on which they do occur. The more frequent this is (the higher the probability of the response), the stronger the response is judged to be.

(2) Extinction. Think back to the person who has become classically conditioned to sweat and tremble when he walks into the dentist's surgery and imagine that he now goes for a long course of dental attention during which he experiences no pain at all. It is probable that the re-

sponses conditioned to the sight and smell of the surgery will lessen and perhaps drop out completely. This process is known as extinction. If the CS is presented on a number of occasions on which the US is repeatedly omitted, i.e. there is no reinforcement, then the CRs diminish.

The time course of extinction follows a remarkably regular pattern. This is shown in the graph below. The main exception to this relatively

Figure 2.1 Extinction

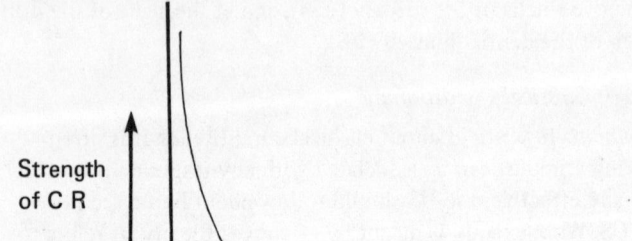

smooth curve of extinction is in the phenomenon known as *spontaneous recovery*. Go back to the example of the man visiting his dentist. He has undergone his course of painless treatment and what we might term his conditioned anxiety has apparently extinguished. Now, a year passes before he walks into the surgery again. At this point some of his CRs will have gained a little in strength, although they will not have returned to their original power. They have recovered spontaneously, simply with the passage of time, no further experiences of CS-US pairing having occurred. Then, of course, if again the US does not occur (i.e. there is no pain), the CR will extinguish again, very rapidly.

(3) Generalisation. Mention was made earlier of the relative ubiquitousness of classical conditioning. From the viewpoint of biological adaptivity it would be inefficient for *every* new classically conditioned response to be acquired in the sometimes lengthy way described above. In fact, classical conditioning is speeded up and extended by generalisation, both at the level of the stimulus and that of the response.

To deal with stimulus generalisation first, imagine that Pavlov's dogs had been conditioned to salivate to the CS of a note on a tuning-fork rather than to a light. Once the response had been firmly established, i.e. was strong, then it would also be made, in diminished strength, to notes on other tuning forks which were near to the first on the musical scale. The more alike is the new note to the original then the more completely it would substitute for it. The more dissimilar it is then the less likely is the response.

Stimulus generalisation can also be well exemplified by the instance of the person who receives painful injections. Not only will he show conditioned anxiety responses to the sight of nurses carrying hypodermic needles, but also to other nurses carrying other objects or even to other people such as ward orderlies wearing uniforms similar to those worn by nurses.

Response generalisation is less common and less important to classical conditioning than is stimulus generalisation and can be dealt with quickly. It simply refers to the likelihood of responses similar to the originally conditioned response being made in the presence of the same CS. For example, if a child has been conditioned the hard way to draw back (CR) his hand from the sight (CS) of a hot fireguard (US) because once or twice he actually touched it and pulled back his hand (UR), then the CR of pulling back his hand is likely to generalise to his other hand and other limbs without further experiences of the US.

(4) Discrimination. If stimulus generalisation in classical conditioning can be summarised as a reaction to similarities, discrimination can be described as its opposite – a reaction to differences. In one of his original experiments, Pavlov trained his dogs to make a CR to the CS of a circle and *not* to make the response to a stimulus of an ellipse – simply by never pairing the ellipse with the US. The animals had been trained to discriminate, a technique which can be used to find out whether or not an animal is *capable* of making particular discriminations.

In a more natural setting it may well be that our hypothetical patient who is still receiving painful injections eventually learns to discriminate between the sight of a nurse carrying a hypodermic needle and one carrying something else. He makes conditioned responses to the former but not to the latter.

As an aside here it is worth noting that once Pavlov had established a discrimination between circles and ellipses, he gradually altered the semi-axes of the ellipses until they approximated more and more to a circle. When the ratio between the semi-axes was 9:8, the dogs behaved as though they had had a breakdown, whimpering, crying, scratching to get out of the apparatus, and ceasing to respond at all. By placing the dogs in a situation where a CS was simultaneously prompting them to respond and not to respond, Pavlov had engendered the first demonstration of what subsequently became known as experimental neurosis. This has been used by those who argue that neuroses are learned.

(5) Higher-order Conditioning. The final important characteristic of classical conditioning is that it can take place at what is termed a higher (or secondary) order. Once a neutral stimulus has acquired the capacity to elicit a conditioned response, i.e. once it has become a conditioned stimulus, in turn it can be linked to another neutral stimulus using the latter as a CS and the original stimulus now having US-like properties. So, for example, if Pavlov's dogs had been trained to salivate to a light and then this light had been closely preceded by a bell, they would have learned to salivate to the bell — even though the bell had never been linked to the US of food. Of course, response strength to the bell would be less, although it would be possible to increase it by exposing the dogs to the sequence:

bell (CS2)--------light (CS1)--------food (US).

Such *chains* of conditioning can become quite lengthy and probably occur often in real life. Through such a chain the person who has developed conditioned anxiety responses to his dentist might eventually make them when he is cleaning his teeth on the morning of his visit to the surgery. The CRs will have been previously linked in a long backward chain from the dentist's chair to the person's bathroom.

Instrumental Conditioning

The Basic Process

Some psychologists argue that instrumental conditioning is concerned with most behaviour of most organisms. It seems to be functional, that is, to involve anything that a person does which has consequences in his environment. In distinction to the respondent, elicited behaviour which characterises classical conditioning, instrumental conditioning involves emitted, operant, apparently voluntary behaviour. It is thought to lie behind what occurs when, for example, children learn to behave in ways thought appropriate by adults, or when adults go out and earn their living, or even when a lion-tamer tames lions.

Although instrumental conditioning has been studied in the laboratory in many ways, it was B.F. Skinner, some 40 years ago, who developed the most far-reaching set of experimental procedures. He devised an operant conditioning chamber, more usually known as a Skinner box, which provided a controlled environment in which to study the acquisition and performance of instrumental behaviour, and which could be adapted for use with many organisms – even man, in some cases.

Since the laboratory rat is the animal which has been most often studied in this context, the description of a rat Skinner box should be sufficient to give the general idea. The details would, of course, differ for different species. It consists literally of a box, about one foot cube, which has solid walls, a grid floor, and on one wall a light, a depressable bar, and a tray into which food can be delivered. The functions of these pieces of apparatus and the behaviour of the rat in the box can be controlled and monitored at long range by electronic or computerised equipment, although this was done by hand originally.

Figure 2.2 Skinner Box or Operant Conditioning Chamber

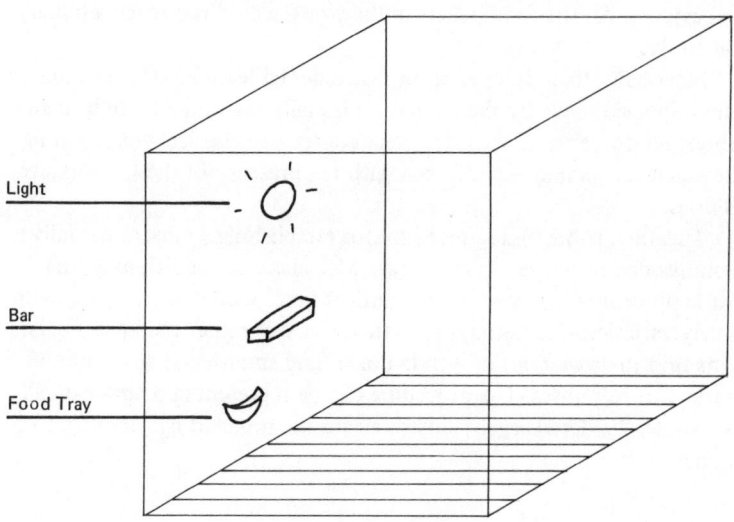

Put into such a box and left alone, a hungry (food-deprived) rat will press the bar occasionally as part of its general exploration. The frequency with which it does this in a given period of time is known as its *operant level.* Having established this, the experimenter then connects the food magazine to the box such that every time the bar is pressed a pellet of food is delivered automatically into the food tray. Typically, the rat notices this and eats it. Soon it is pressing the bar and eating the food pellets quite frequently. The food is said to have *reinforced* the bar-pressing, learning necessarily having occurred since the rat is pressing the bar far more frequently than it did when its operant level was measured. In general, a record of rate of responses against time gives a measure of the course of operant or instrumental conditioning.

Occasionally an experimenter is faced with what seems to be a recalcitrant rat; one which never seems to press the bar. Of course, if the bar is never pressed (i.e. the desired behaviour never emitted) the animal cannot be reinforced for it and will never learn or be conditioned. The experimenter then *shapes* the rat. This simply involves watching the rat closely and delivering a pellet of food for successive approximations to bar-pressing. So the food is used to reinforce a series of graded responses which to begin with might merely involve a movement towards the bar but which will always end in pressing. For instrumental conditioning to occur the behaviour (responses) involved must either happen naturally to begin with or at least be part of an organism's potential repertoire of behaviours. All the food pellets in the world would not teach a hungry rat to fly.

Essentially then, in operant or instrumental learning or conditioning, the responses made by the animal are literally instrumental in bringing about reinforcement. This is in clear contrast to classical conditioning in which the animal is reinforced with the presence of the US whatever it does.

This then is the basic procedure for establishing an instrumentally conditioned response. As is the case with classical conditioning, the basic procedure has been used countless times with many species, with many variations (sometimes the rats run mazes rather than press bars, or cats find their way out of puzzle boxes, and so on), and an enormous variety of responses. The procedure can be represented diagramatically as below, the details again illustrated for the moment by recourse to a hungry rat.

S1	R1	S2	R2
CS	CR	US (reinforcing stimulus)	UR
Bar	Pressing	Food	Eating

This representation emphasises two important points. First, the US or reinforcing stimulus *only* occurs if the conditioned response is made. And second, unlike classical conditioning, the conditioned and unconditioned responses in instrumental conditioning are quite dissimilar.

To define instrumental conditioning: Instrumental (operant) conditioning is the strengthening of a stimulus-response association by following the response with a reinforcing stimulus.

Note that in instrumental conditioning the reinforcing stimulus has no effect on the conditioned response at the time it occurs; it cannot, the response is already past. It simply alters the *future* likelihood of that response. Depending on the nature of the reinforcer (see below) it makes the preceding, conditioned response either more or less likely to occur, it *strengthens or weakens* it.

The examples of instrumental conditioning in real life are legion, and very little different from rats in boxes. For the moment, consider just two. First, if a child in a classroom raises his hand and asks a question and before answering the teacher smiles at him and tells him what a good question it was, he will be more likely to raise his hand and ask questions in the future. The smile and verbal praise have reinforced his behaviour, that is, they have increased its future probability. Second, if on occasion you idly put your hand down the side of a settee or chair and by chance find a coin, you will be for ever reaching down the side of furniture. Your behaviour has been reinforced. It might seem that this is just behaving sensibly; it is obvious that you try again in a place in which you have once found money. This is so; much of instrumental behaviour and learning consists of what in everyday terms would be called good sense. However, it is not always so.

The Phenomena of Instrumental Conditioning

(1) Measurement. As mentioned above, the main way of assessing the strength of an instrumentally conditioned response is by looking at its *rate*. In general, the more responses that occur within a given time period then the stronger the response is judged to be. This is simply another way of deciding how probable it is that the response occurs at all; the greater the probability the stronger the response.

Similarly, an indication of response strength comes from the *size* or force of the response; if it is performed vigorously it is judged to be stronger. Also, it is so judged if it occurs quickly, a measure known as response *latency*. It will be remembered that these measures of response strength are very similar to those taken in classical conditioning.

(2) Extinction. Not only does the phenomenon of extinction occur in

instrumental conditioning, it also provides the final measure of the strength of the conditioned response. Think back to the child who has been reinforced for asking a question in class. Now, if every time he raises his hand the teacher ignores him he will gradually stop raising his hand. The response has extinguished because it has ceased to be followed by the reinforcing stimulus, the time course of this process being very similar to that which is shown in classical conditioning.

Conditioned responses vary as to how *resistant* they are to extinction. The more resistant they are, the longer they last without reinforcement, the stronger they are judged to be or to have been. Many other facets of instrumental conditioning affect response strength; it will be returned to frequently.

(3) Amount, Number and Timing of Reinforcements. In considering instrumental conditioning it is important to make a distinction between learning and performance, i.e. between how a new response is learned and then how well it is performed once it has been acquired. For example, starting from scratch I might learn to play tennis of a reasonable standard quite quickly, but on certain days still perform very poorly. This poor performance might have very little to do with the original learning. The problem involved in this distinction is seen more obviously when amount of reinforcement is considered. Not surprisingly, the amount of reinforcement affects learning – up to a point. If you write an article for a newspaper and are paid £100 for it you are more likely to write another than if you were paid only £1. However, amount of reinforcement affects both learning and performance. Again, up to a point, the larger the reinforcement the more effective the learning, and also once learning has taken place, performance is sometimes more effective with larger rewards.

Also important are numbers of reinforcements and their timing. Up to a point, the strength of an instrumental response increases with the number of reinforcements it leads to, and response strength is built up faster (learning occurs more efficiently) the less time intervenes between the response and the reinforcement. Hence, if you wish to strengthen (make more probable) a generous act by a child, it is better to reinforce it straight away than to wait until later. (Several times in this analysis, statements have been qualified by saying 'up to a point'. The reasons for these qualifications will become clear later.)

(4) Generalisation and Discrimination. Just as in classical conditioning, both stimulus and response generalisation occur in instrumental condi-

tioning, again with important biological utility attendant on them. Each
new response does not have to be laboriously learned. Think of the rat
pressing the bar in the Skinner box for food reinforcement; if he is put
into a similar box with a similar bar he will be likely to press it – stimulus generalisation. If a very young child is reinforced for calling his
father 'Daddy', he may well spend some time calling all men 'Daddy' –
a case of inappropriate stimulus generalisation.

Going back to the rat in the box, he may well press the bar with
either or both of his forepaws or even with his nose – response generalisation. At the everyday level, we do not have to learn to make social
responses to every new person that we meet and the social responses we
make can take various forms and be expressed in various ways. Both
stimulus and response generalisation considerably broaden the scope of
instrumental learning and make it far less of an arduous process than it
might at first appear.

When thinking of the nature of discrimination in instrumental conditioning, yet another type of stimulus has to be introduced – a *discriminative stimulus*; it emphasises the opposed nature of generalisation and
discrimination. Imagine again a hungry rat which has learned to press a
bar in a Skinner box. If the experimenter were drastically to change the
size, shape and colour of the walls of the box then it is likely that the
rat would no longer press the bar. The original characteristics of the box
have set the scene for making the response – they have acted as discriminative stimuli. Think of the difficulties some people experience when
for some reason their favourite chair is usurped; they cannot perform
their normal instrumental responses as well as usual.

A rat, or indeed any organism, can be trained to make instrumental
responses in the presence of some stimuli but not in the presence of
others, to press a bar when a light is on but not when it is off, for
example. Not only does an animal make such discriminations but, like
classical conditioning, instrumental conditioning can also be used to
determine what discriminations it can make. In this way it can be determined whether or not an animal has colour vision for example.

To conclude with an everyday example, there are an enormous
number of discriminations that anyone makes when driving a car. For
instance, road signs set the scene for a variety of instrumental driving
responses representing the general rules of the road.

(5) Higher-order Conditioning. Another parallel between classical and
instrumental conditioning is that higher-order conditioning can occur in
both, long chains of learning being formed in this way. This secondary

conditioning also links in with discriminative stimuli, for it is these which also sometimes act as secondary reinforcers. Back again to the rat in the box. Now, it has learned to press the bar and every time it does so a light comes on. However, by making the food magazine inoperative, the response has nearly extinguished, but in the dark. Then, the light is reconnected such that if and when the rat presses the bar the light comes on even though no food clicks down into the tray. The rat's rate of bar-pressing increases rapidly for a while. Through association with what is called the *primary* (unlearned, built-in) reinforcer of food, the light has taken on its own (secondary; learned) reinforcing properties.

With these rather complex ideas it may seem that the problems of everyday life are far away. This is not so for the very good reason that under some conditions a secondary or learned reinforcer can influence responses other than those originally learned. This greatly increases the possible range and flexibility of learning. Probably the most powerful example of this comes from a child's early relationship with his mother.

To begin with a mother is not a primary reinforcer for her child; rather, she is a source of such reinforcement, mainly in the form of food and also perhaps warmth and comfort. This extreme dependence of the child on his mother promotes virtually all of the child's initial learning. Whenever an infant receives a basic primary reinforcer such as food, he is with his mother. Not only is she a discriminative stimulus for all manner of instrumental responses, she is also strongly associated with primary reinforcement. Through this association she acquires enormous power as a secondary reinforcer. So powerful is she in being able to promote new learning that she eventually has the virtual status of a primary reinforcer herself. Her very presence and of course her approval and affection can reinforce an abundance of new instrumental responses in her child.

The importance of this almost inevitable capacity in a mother is clearly of immense importance for the learning of a very wide range of behaviours in the young child, especially allowing for the development of his social responses. When the ideas of stimulus and response generalisation are added in as well, the ramifications are tremendous. Responses made to the mother as a secondary reinforcer also tend to be made to other people and the real beginnings of social behaviour are seen; this of course being especially important to human beings.

In passing, it should be noted that there do not appear to be very many primary reinforcers; those which are genetically or biologically determined. These are restricted to the basic necessities of life, such as food, water, oxygen, etc. with the possible addition of sex and one of a somewhat different status — the avoidance of pain. All other reinforcers are believed to be secondary, or learned, in association with the primary reinforcers. Later, in adult life, from some points of view, such secondary reinforcers seem of more importance than primary reinforcers. For example, social approval and money are very powerful sources of reinforcement for adult instrumental behaviour.

(6) Partial Reinforcement. So far the way in which instrumental conditioning has been described gives the slightly misleading impression that either in real life or in the laboratory, *every* response is reinforced, i.e. that reinforcement is continuous. Of course, this is not so. It is rare to find the situation that every time a response is made it is reinforced; reinforcement usually occurs only on occasion. This is described as partial or intermittent reinforcement.

Reinforcement for instrumental responding can occur intermittently in four basic ways, these being known as the main *schedules of reinforcement*. They are outlined in the table below.

Schedules of Partial Reinforcement

Time based	*Response based*
Fixed intervals	Fixed ratios
Variable intervals	Variable ratios

To start with the time based schedules, it happens that some reinforcements are received only after particular periods of time. These might be fixed, at exactly every 30 seconds or every 30 minutes for example, or might occur on average at every 30 seconds or 30 minutes. Respectively these refer to fixed and variable intervals. Such schedules imply that if the organism makes at least one of the necessary responses during the particular time period then he will receive reinforcement, and if he makes no responses of course he will receive no reinforcement. Alternatively, if he makes more than one response within the time interval he will still receive only one reinforcement.

Response based schedules of reinforcement depend on the ratio between responses and reinforcement. For example, a rat in a box might be reinforced only for every fifth or every twentieth bar press that it makes, or possibly for every fifth or twentieth response on average. As with interval schedules, these refer to fixed and variable ratios respectively.

Once again, this very academic sort of analysis may seem a long way from real life. In fact, it is not, since most of our everyday behaviour is reinforced only intermittently. Two examples will suffice. A person at work whose payment is linked to the number of items he produces is functioning on a ratio schedule of reinforcement. So, for every 1,000 double-headed, cross-threaded screws he makes he receives £1. Similarly, a mother who gives her son a hug and kiss and tells him how good he has been a few times each day is reinforcing many different aspects of his behaviour on a series of variable interval schedules of reinforcement.

Partial reinforcement has a very special effect on instrumentally conditioned responses. It makes the responses stronger than they would have been had they been reinforced every time they occurred. That is, it ensures that the responses are made at a higher rate and that they take far longer to extinguish when the reinforcement is no longer available. This characteristic has an obvious importance in day-to-day learning. The sheer complexity of life makes it impossible for reinforcers to be constantly available. A mother cannot always be there to say 'good boy' to her child, a teacher cannot praise every good bit of work, a person being trained to use an artificial limb cannot be encouraged for every movement. This is all to the good. The responses are being learned and performed *more* strongly by being reinforced only some of the time. The theoretical reasons for this are very complex and need not be of concern here. It is simply a very useful fact of life.

(7) Types of Instrumental Conditioning. Throughout this discussion the only examples of instrumental conditioning have involved positive reinforcement, events which act directly to strengthen behaviour; for whatever reason they are pleasant to the individual. However, some types of stimuli are unpleasant, either inherently or due to learned associations with other unpleasant stimuli. This leads to a variety of types of instrumental conditioning, other than that in which behaviour is strengthened by positive reinforcers.

First, and most obvious, we learn to *escape* from aversive, harmful stimuli. A child who sticks his finger into a light socket and gets an electric shock will probably not do it again too readily. He has escaped from the shock by pulling out his finger and has learned to *avoid* the likelihood of it happening again. He has learned to keep his hands away from light sockets.

In psychological laboratories, avoidance conditioning is often studied in what is called a shuttle-box. This is a box with two compartments separated by a hurdle. An animal is placed in one compartment; a stimulus such as a light is presented to him for a fixed period of time and then the animal is given a noxious stimulus such as an electric shock to the feet. He can escape this by jumping over the hurdle into the second compartment. Or he can avoid it altogether if he learns to jump when the light comes on, but before the shock is delivered. This apparatus and procedure simply provides a means of studying a very common process. All of us have learned to make very many avoidance responses and do so every day of our lives when the occasion demands. The sound of a car horn makes us jump to safety and the sight of a certain person coming towards us on the street leads us to cross to the other side to avoid a conversation which we believe will be unpleasant.

A Skinner box can also be used to study avoidance behaviour. It simply involves an animal in learning to press the bar whilst a light is on but before a shock is given to him. If he does so then the shock is postponed for a certain time period. What is interesting about avoidance learning is that a negative stimulus is being used to *strengthen* behaviour.

Of equal importance in normal life is *punishment.* Unpleasant stimuli not only function to promote avoidance responses, but also act as punishers of whatever behaviour immediately precedes them. In general, in a similar way to which a positive stimulus strengthens immediately preceding behaviour, so a negative stimulus will weaken it. Once again, everyday life abounds in punishment, from the 'natural' outcomes of the pain involved in breaking a limb through a fall from a stupidly ridden bicycle, through the slap of a mother's hand when her child is rude, to the institutionalised punishment of imprisonment for illegal acts.

It is clear that punishment does alter instrumental behaviour, but its effects are by no means as obvious as those of reward. Either occurring naturally or being used manipulatively, the effects of punishment are to lessen the likelihood of some disadvantageous or undesirable behaviour. But the main problem is that even though a stimulus might *appear* to be unpleasant it does not necessarily follow that it will be effective as a punisher (to a limited extent the same is true of reinforcers – one man's meat may be another's poison). To chastise a child for talking in class may well have the effect of making him *more* likely to talk – the chastisement is a form of attention and this can be reinforcing. Sometimes a person who punishes another is so upset by this that he follows the punishment with a great show of affection. The punished person is then instrumentally conditioned to behave in certain ways that lead to the mild punishment followed by the larger reward.

In dealing with these and similar problems of punishment, Church (1963) and Azrin and Holz (1966) variously conclude that behaviour is most suppressed when the punishment is associated with it directly, both in place and time. Even so, the use of punishment in learning carries certain disadvantages.

(a) Punishment makes no positive prescriptions for behaviour; it merely says 'don't do this'.

(b) Punishment may well make a person withdraw from the situation entirely, perhaps expressing hatred or anxiety.

(c) Sometimes apparent punishment can become rewarding.

As will be seen in more detail in the next chapter, punishment is used in attempts to control behaviour, behavioural control being the other side of the coin to conditioning and learning. In using punishment manipulatively to change a person's behaviour it is worth bearing in mind the following points.

(a) It is better (more effective) to reinforce appropriate responses if this is at all possible.

(b) If punishment is used, then it is best to combine it with positive reinforcement.

(c) It is possible to use *mild* punishment informatively, that is, just to let a person know that he is on the wrong track – frown rather than a slap.

(d) Serious thought should be given to the appropriateness of punishment with very young children. They tend to overgeneralise rather than discriminate and therefore learn undesirable things from too much punishment. Too much behaviour might be suppressed.

(e) If punishment is used at all then it should be associated very clearly with the undesired behaviour and with nothing else.

(f) Punishment should be administered instantly rather than later. This point has obvious implications about the inevitably long gaps which intervene between crime and punishment in most societies.

Problems and Theories

One of the basic problems of instrumental conditioning is that of delineating just to how much of the massive range of human learning it applies. Some psychologists would argue that, together with classical conditioning, it accounts for all human learning. Others maintain that it is impossible to account for the more complex forms of learning with models of simple conditioning. Conditioning seems to be too automatic and to have no room for (necessary) concepts such as understanding and insight.

One instance will exemplify the problem. As long ago as 1925, Kohler carried out a study in which he put a chimpanzee in a cage and gave it a short stick. Outside the cage and out of reach of the stick was a banana. Also outside the cage, but within reach of the short stick was a longer stick. After a few ineffectual attempts to reach the banana with the short stick, Kohler's chimps gave up and appeared to 'think' about the problem for some time. Then they made the obvious (to us) response of drawing in the long stick with the short one and using the former to draw in the banana. Kohler believed this to demonstrate insight learning, a very complex cognitive capacity. But could such behaviour be accounted for by a long chain of conditioning and past experience? There is no simple answer to this and to many similar questions about human learning. However, the more complex forms of learning will be returned to in the chapter after next.

The division between what might be called behavioural and cognitive approaches is also reflected in the two very different types of theory of learning which psychologists have devised. Here is not the place to go into these in great detail, but a very brief overview might be instructive.

There is a long tradition of what are termed stimulus-response (S-R) theories of learning. The essential assumption of these theories is that stimuli and responses are linked through associations and/or reinforcement and learning is responsible for forging this link. Such theories always emphasise behavioural responses and deal with long chains of simple elements. They say little, if anything, about any central mechanisms which might be involved in learning, either physiologically or cognitively. Probably the best known S-R learning theory is that of Hull (1943) whose basic hypothesis was that $E = H \times D$.

E refers to output potential or performance, H refers to habit strength or learning, and D refers to drive or motivation. Thus in Hull's very influential view, performance depends on how well an activity is learned and how highly the individual is motivated, learning (H) increasing with the number of reinforced responses, and motivation (D) with increasing deprivation of the necessary objects, such as food.

The cognitive learning theorists naturally deal with the same set of facts as the S-R theorists, but they put a very different interpretation on them, emphasising central rather than peripheral processes. So, an S-R theorist might say that a man has a meal in a restaurant because he is pulled there by a long chain of learned connections between muscular stimuli and responses. Alternatively, a cognitive theorist might argue that the man goes to the restaurant with the *purpose* of having a meal, or because he *expects* to eat. In other words, he accounts for learning by speculating about cognitive or mental concepts such as expectancies. It is still open to question which of these two approaches is the more fruitful or which provides the better theory.

To complete this description of conditioning it is important to mention two further problems which psychologists have not yet solved satisfactorily. The first concerns the nature of reinforcement and reinforcers. How is it possible to decide whether or not a particular stimulus is a reinforcer? In answer, one cannot say that it is a stimulus which strengthens behaviour, since this would be circular. The behaviour would be undefined independently of the reinforcer and the reinforcer undefined independently of the behaviour. It would be like saying that a man goes to a restaurant because he is reinforced with the food he has there, and that we know that the food is a reinforcer because the man goes to the restaurant to get it. The only way to break this circle is to show that a stimulus can act as a reinforcer for a variety of behaviours under many conditions. But this is not always easy to do, particularly since what is reinforcing for one person might not be for the next. Jack Sprat could eat no fat, his wife could eat no lean.

The final problem concerns the relationship between classical and instrumental conditioning. In this chapter they have been described as though they were quite distinct processes, and indeed psychologists have devised procedures to study them quite separately. However, in everyday life they are not so distinct, most learning probably involving a mixture of the two. In making any analysis of everyday learning or of training procedures it is worth bearing in mind this point. For example, if a person is learning to ride a bicycle he is reinforced for the instrumental responses he makes both by managing to stay upright and move about and also by external encouragement from his friends and family. However, he will also have moments when he falls or nearly falls off, this reflexively pumping adrenalin round his body and arousing him generally. Linked to these physiological responses in time will be the sight, sound, and feel of the bicycle. To begin with then he will have been classically conditioned to make these physiological responses to otherwise neutral stimuli. It often seems that classical conditioning is concerned with the more emotional responses and instrumental conditioning with the more non-emotional or perhaps functional responses. And of course many aspects of everyday life have their emotional and non-emotional aspects.

Summary Points

(1) Learning is a process which determines any relatively permanent changes that occur in behaviour; it involves the acquisition of new connections between stimuli and responses. Theories about this process either dwell on the external S-R level or are concerned with possible cognitive structures such as expectancies.

(2) The simplest forms of learning are classical and instrumental conditioning, each of these involving two types of stimuli (USs and CSs) and two types of response (URs and CRs). They account for much (if not all) of the learning of everyone. Various techniques and procedures have been developed to measure and study the two types of conditioning.

(3) The basic phenomena of classical and instrumental conditioning are: acquisition, extinction, generalisation, discrimination, higher-order or secondary conditioning, and partial reinforcement.

(4) The basic principles of conditioning are association and reinforcement, there being particular problems associated with the latter, and with its converse, punishment.

(5) The timing, place and type of reinforcement and punishment all have important influences on learning.

(6) Conditioning is not only studied in the laboratory. It occurs naturally all the time, both types of conditioning usually being involved in any learning. Also, the principles of conditioning can be seen at work whenever one person attempts to teach or train another, and even in the way in which society's institutions (such as the law) are constructed.

Study Questions – 2

(1) Describe classical and instrumental conditioning using examples from a hospital setting. Make clear what are the USs, CSs, URs, and CRs.

(2) What do you think would be more effective for recovery, encouraging a patient *every* time he engaged in self-help behaviour or only some of the time?

(3) Are there any circumstances in your profession in which you would punish a patient? (Be careful in your definition of punishment.) If society were to permit it, do you think punishment could be more widely used in hospitals as an effective way to control behaviour?

(4) From what you know of patients and of your colleagues, attempt to illustrate the adage that 'one man's meat is another man's poison'. Why do you think that this holds true and why is it important to conditioning?

(5) How would you train someone to: ride a bicycle; type; improve his handwriting; write with the other hand; be more generous; swear less; smile more often?

(6) Do you think that your patients learn anything that cannot be explained by simple classical and instrumental conditioning? If so, what is it and how would you explain it?

(7) In your course and amongst your patients some people learn (or condition) faster than others. Why do you think this is? (Bear in mind that the answer is almost certainly *not* just a matter of intelligence.)

(8) Whether consciously or not, there must have been many instances in which you have conditioned or taught patients or in which they have conditioned or taught you. From among such examples consider some of the ways in which learning or conditioning might go wrong.

(9) Do you think that you could condition any of your patients to do anything? What would set the limits on such conditioning? Would the same limits obtain outside a hospital?

(10) In your opinion can people be conditioned without them being aware that it is happening? Has it ever happened to you and you have found out later? Has your awareness had any effect on your subsequent behaviour?

3 BEHAVIOUR MODIFICATION

The last chapter was concerned with the ways in which conditioning (simple learning) occurs in real life and how it has been studied in the laboratory. If people learn or become conditioned then of course they can be taught; conscious efforts can be made to condition them. This is the other side of the coin. There is nothing sinister about the idea of conditioning people. All of us do it every day of our lives, although perhaps not consciously. Be this as it may, the general principles of conditioning have been systematically applied in many ways; these range from the development of teaching machines to brain-washing and indoctrination — the application of conditioning does have its sinister aspects.

In the present chapter the aim is to concentrate on what is arguably the most interesting of the applications of conditioning, namely to medical problems, particularly where these concern abnormal behaviour. This area of applied research and practical techniques has come to be known as behaviour modification.

As might be expected of an approach to abnormality which comes from a very objective tradition, behaviour modification focuses precisely on behaviour which can be defined clearly, and observed and measured. Faced with what is normally termed a mental disorder, the behaviour modifier asks three basic questions.
(1) What aspects of the person's behaviour are maladaptive? That is, if the person is described as neurotic for example, what does he actually *do* that can be regarded as harmful to himself or to others?
(2) What is there in the individual's environment that supports the behaviour in question? Of course, from a conditioning point of view behaviour would simply extinguish if it were not supported by reinforcing stimuli. What are these?
(3) What in the individual's environment can be changed in order to change the maladaptive behaviour? Again, in terms of conditioning, it is only via changes in the environment that some behaviour will disappear and other behaviour will take its place.

To summarise the standpoint taken by the behaviour modifier, if for example he is told that a person has an ego which needs strengthening, he asks what this means in terms of what the person does and how it shows up in his interaction with the environment.

Before going into more detail about the aims and the techniques of behaviour modification, it is important to point out its main and very far-reaching assumption, since this has implications for the way in which mental disorder in general is dealt with. The assumption is that abnormal behaviour may be defined as *learned habits* which are bad for the individual, and not that he is in some way mentally diseased. This then is throwing aside the traditional medical model of abnormality. Of course, this model is so much a part of everyday discourse that it is often forgotten that it represents only one (arbitrary) way of looking at things; it is just a model.

The medical model of abnormality has it that any behaviour which might be involved is superficial; it is merely 'symptomatic' of something deeper, this something being the actual abnormality. So the search is made for the underlying causes of the behavioural symptoms. Also, it is assumed that it is worthless to deal solely with the behaviour because the roots of what is wrong would not be laid bare; the 'real' trouble would not have been dealt with. On the other hand, the behavioural model of abnormality takes the standpoint that it is a matter of habits rather than diseases. If the habits are changed then the abnormality has been dealt with; it is a question of interaction between behaviour and environment.

At present, which of these two viewpoints is correct, if indeed either of them is, remains unresolved. Ultimately, it is an empirical question and so the immediate reaction is one of expediency. One can ask which of the two models generates better therapeutic outcomes for people with problems. The evidence gathered in answer to this question points in more than one direction, largely depending on the nature of the abnormality. However, this is a digression. The important point to bear in mind is that the remainder of this chapter is based on a behavioural or conditioning and learning model of abnormality or mental disorder.

Maladaptive Behaviour

Since the learning theory view is that maladaptive behaviours are learned and maintained in just the same way as are adaptive behaviours, the implication is that there is no discontinuity between the normal and the abnormal, the healthy and the sick. What then is the difference between the two? The argument is that any society has expectations concerning what is acceptable behaviour in its members, acceptable that is within the family and in society at large. And society has developed its reinforcers for these behaviours – attention, affection, money, medals, etc. In this context, maladaptive behaviour is that which is *thought* to be inappropriate by the important people in one's life, that is by those who control the reinforcers. Thus it is parents who judge whether or not a child's behaviour is maladaptive and it is family, friends, colleagues and employers who judge an adult's behaviour, and in some cases even the person himself might make the judgement.

The main implication of this view is that ideas of what is abnormal will change from place to place and from time to time. Conceptions of abnormality will differ between societies (as indeed they do), and even within a society. Also, they might change from one generation to the next, the changing view of neurosis in western society in the last 20 or 30 years perhaps providing an example of this.

The behavioural way of defining maladaptivity and hence mental disorder, raises immediate questions about the regularities which are traditionally seen in those who are classified as mentally ill — even about the division between neurosis and psychosis for example. If it is all a matter of individual learning where do these regularities come from? Each case should be quite distinct from the next. In reply to this implicit criticism, the behaviour modifier or therapist usually makes a number of related points, all of which have some substance.
(1) Classifications of the mentally ill do not in fact show very much in the way of regularity.
(2) There is dissension amongst those that classify — mainly the psychiatrists.
(3) There are vogue ways of thinking which influence judgements and which lead to much pressure to actually classify people according to the regular symptoms which are laid out in the text books.
(4) Within a hospital there are strong pressures for the inmate to adopt 'conventional' roles, particularly that of being docile and non-troublesome. In fact, nurses and attendants command a large number of powerful reinforcers which maintain such behaviour. Anyone who has spent some time in any institution knows of the massive importance of small privileges and threats of punishment. The general point, then, is that the behaviour modifier has convincing arguments that the regularities found in classifications of the mentally ill might sometimes be spurious.

Causes and Maintenance of Maladaptive Behaviour

Although those who make a conditioning-based analysis of abnormal behaviour do not look much further than at the behaviour itself, they still have to consider how it comes about. In so doing their suggestions are very reminiscent of some of the basic phenomena of conditioning described in the last chapter. For example, any behaviour which lessens the likelihood of aversive stimuli is positively reinforcing and is therefore likely to occur again. This is the precise way of saying that we learn to avoid things which are unpleasant to us. In real life, this means that we learn to avoid people or situations or even behaviour that have been associated with unpleasant stimuli. Then generalisation may occur, so that a person may not be able to distinguish between people or situations that are beneficial or pleasant and those which are not. This could lead to what has been termed general anxiety, a condition basic to most neuroses.

A second possible way in which maladaptive behaviour is developed is that adaptive responses are simply not learned. Consider, for example, a person who is socially withdrawn and isolated as a child. He will have had very little opportunity to have practised or to have learned or to have been reinforced for developing social skills. This leads to the development of a vicious circle. Future social situations are unrewarding and so there is even less chance for practice, and so on.

To take another example, maladaptive behaviours may be learned directly through instrumental conditioning; a person may even be positively reinforced for them. Think for instance of the behaviour of most people when they are confronted with someone who stutters. They very often pay far more attention to him when he hesitates in his speech than when he does not. They might well be effectively reinforcing him for stuttering. But of course, socially, it is very difficult to do otherwise than this.

Finally, there is the more extreme type of emotional reaction which can result from various experiences with learning. For example, it is argued by some applied learning theorists that pathological depression may result from the simultaneous removal from a person of a series of very important reinforcers, such as when a loved one dies or he loses his job.

In general, it can be seen that it is possible to account for the development of any type of abnormal or maladaptive behaviour from a conditioning or learning standpoint. Whether it is appropriate so to do is beyond the scope of this discussion. The important point is that this approach brings with it a number of practical techniques which are of probable help in dealing with behaviour problems.

Before going on to describe some of these techniques, a final word should be said about how maladaptive behaviour is maintained once it has developed. The broad answer is that it is maintained by reinforcement, although the reinforcer may be different from that which was effective in its development. From the principles of conditioning it follows quite clearly that no behaviour which is unreinforced will continue; it simply extinguishes.

Take just one very commonplace example. Think of a person who relatively early in life shares a room with someone who snores. To combat this he learns to go to sleep with his head under the pillow. The pillow over the ear is associated with the basic reinforcement of going to sleep and so becomes a discriminative stimulus for sleeping. Years later the room-mate has gone but the pillow remains. This is only a very mild form of maladaptive behaviour but the same principles could well be at work in more extreme cases. For example, a child might learn to switch off his attention because his parents always nag and deride him. As an adult, his parents are no longer so important to him but he may have generalised so that any social event is an occasion to switch off. This would be clearly maladaptive and could even look like the beginnings of the social withdrawal and detachment that characterises schizophrenia.

Methods of Behaviour Change

As might be expected from the previous chapter, there are two principal schools of methods of behavioural change — one uses instrumental conditioning and is expressed in Skinnerian terms and the other classical conditioning and Pavlovian terms. From these schools a large number of techniques have been developed, although not very many principles are involved. Those that are can be summarised as: the systematic use of environmental contingencies to alter a person's responses to stimuli.

Two of the words in this definition stand out above the others. Most importantly, behaviour modification is *systematic*. All of us modify one another's behaviour every day, but we do it haphazardly. In dealing with abnormal behaviour the behaviour therapist works consciously and systematically with a particular end in view.

Second, *responses* are involved, not just a specific response. So the good behaviour modifier will not only get rid of the maladaptive behaviour but will replace it with more appropriate behaviours. It is not that the extinguished behaviour will be replaced by a vacuum — a behavioural vacuum is impossible. Rather, it is that if the behaviour modifier does not replace it with something appropriate, another maladaptive response might take its place. As far as possible, nothing is left to chance.

What follows is not an exhaustive list of methods of behavioural change. The examples have been chosen to be representative of the many techniques which have been devised.

(1) Assertive Responses

Wolpe (1958) who has been an influential behaviour therapist was the first to suggest that anxiety and the expression of resentment are incompatible. If a person can be trained to assert himself, then his anxiety should be inhibited. In doing this, the therapist points out to the patient the irrationality of his fears and encourages him to be assertive and to 'insist on his rights'. Sometimes he will set up a series of progressively more difficult social tasks for the person to undertake, first in his imagination and then, as he gains confidence, in real life.

(2) Sexual Responses

Unfortunately many people learn maladaptive sexual behaviour. One way of dealing with some examples of this again involves a graded series of problems. The person is instructed to engage only in those sexual acts which he has a definite desire to perform and which he does not find aversive. Of course, this will usually require the assistance of a willing partner. Then, having had some sexual behaviour associated with positive reinforcement, the person is given a series of tasks, if that is the right word in this context, which approximate more and more to normal sexual behaviour. At this stage the progression towards normality is usually helped by the occurrence of generalisation.

(3) Relaxation

A similar technique to the above is seen with relaxation responses; it has received a very wide application. It began with Jacobson's (1964) idea that a state of relaxation is incompatible with anxiety which is characterised by muscle tension. The anxious patient is taught to relax more and more deeply and the relaxed state is associated with an imagined series of threatening experiences running from the least to the most disturbing. As soon as the patient starts to become tense and anxious he is taken back gently to a less threatening part of the imagined hierarchy. Then, again relaxed, he is slowly taken forward once more.

From the imagined experiences the patient is taken on to a series of real situations in the same slow and gentle progression. Thus a positive reinforcer (relaxation) has been developed for the patient and has been systematically related to experiences which would normally make the patient anxious. This technique, which has enjoyed wide success with some forms of neurosis, is known as systematic desensitisation.

(4) Modelling

A very different technique from relaxation but one which is culled very obviously from everyday life is modelling, in which another person makes and is reinforced for whatever response is to be learned by the patient. The latter is, of course, in a position to observe the other person making the response and being reinforced for it. If the conditions are right the patient will imitate the model's behaviour much as a child imitates the behaviour of a parent or of anyone that he admires. The idea of this type of behaviour modification is that whatever is the stimulus for the maladaptive behaviour is put into a new and more favourable context, and the behaviour of others may serve as a discriminative stimulus for appropriate behaviours from the person with difficulties.

(5) Extinction

An obvious way to modify maladaptive behaviour is simply to extinguish it, although in the complexities of everyday life, this is not always possible. Thinking back to the previous chapter, extinction just involves the removal of whatever reinforcing stimulus is controlling the behaviour. The behaviour is then likely to be reduced in frequency and new behaviour will take its place. If the new behaviour is deemed to be appropriate and useful to the person then it can in turn be reinforced.

The problem with this very straightforward and obvious way of modifying behaviour is that when the behaviour is problematic it is sometimes difficult to determine exactly what is reinforcing it. Also, it is sometimes not possible to remove the reinforcers when they are identified. This is especially so if they come from a person's family or from his job. It may be quite impracticable to lift the individual entirely from his environment, particularly if afterwards he has to return to it.

(6) Positive Reinforcement

Positive reinforcement needs no elucidation. It is the prime technique of behaviour modification and it is used whenever possible. It simply involves the reinforcing of desired rather than maladaptive behaviours. But for it to be used the behaviours must first occur naturally and there must be some stimuli which can be identified as potentially reinforcing to the particular person in his particular circumstances. These are by no means always easy to find.

(7) Satiation

Finally, a rather interesting technique involves making a reinforcing stimulus so abundant that the person becomes full of it and it loses its effectiveness as a reinforcer. It will no longer promote or maintain behaviour. It is rather like what happens if a young child is allowed a bout of unlimited ice-cream or chocolate. He tends to eat himself sick and then not be able to face the food again for some time. Having so demolished one reinforcer, others can be built up in its place and used for more appropriate behaviours.

Case Studies

The techniques described above may all seem a little sterile and academic. The aim of this section is to bring some of them to life a little by describing three case studies in which they, and similar techniques, were used. The cases were chosen from the earlier literature on behaviour modification since they represent a wide variety of possibilities in dealing with very different types of disorder. They embody many of the points made above, particularly in their constant reference to behaviour rather than to speculation about possible underlying dynamic forces.

Case 1: Verbal Behaviour in a Schizophrenic (Isaacs, Thomas & Goldiamond, 1960)

The patient in this case was an impassive schizophrenic who was extremely withdrawn and who had remained mute for some 21 years. Little had been or could be done for him other than to sit him in group therapy sessions with other more outgoing schizophrenics. This did little. On one such occasion the experimenter accidentally dropped a packet of chewing-gum to the floor and as he did so noticed that the patient's eyes momentarily followed its passage. The experimenter therefore decided to try to use chewing-gum as a reinforcer to shape the patient's behaviour (he had at least been transiently interested in it) and determined to meet with him three times per week, individually.

During the first two weeks the experimenter held a stick of gum in front of the patient's face and waited until his gaze turned towards it; when it did he immediately gave him the gum. Soon the patient's eyes would move towards the gum the moment it was held up. In weeks three and four, the experimenter held the gum in the same way, but did not give it to the patient until his eyes moved towards it *and* there was a spontaneous movement of the lips. By the end of the third week there were lip and eye movements. Then, in the fourth week the gum was withheld until there were eye and lip movements and any sort of vocalisation. To begin with this was just a croaking sound.

During the fifth and sixth weeks the experimenter held up the gum and said 'say gum-gum' and giving the gum was made dependent on more and more accurate approximations to this. At the end of the sixth week the patient spontaneously said, 'Gum please' and thereafter would speak, answer questions about his name, age and so on. After this break-through the patient would respond to the experimenter in a wider and wider variety of settings, but to no one else. So by a similar laborious process of shaping, the patient's verbal responses were made to generalise to other people.

These rather dramatic results with someone who had not spoken for many years illustrate many points. First, they were achieved relatively quickly and with only positive reinforcement being used. But this was only possible once the appropriate reinforcer had been found. Very often the finding of a good reinforcer is difficult and as in this case depends on a mixture of luck and keen observation.

Further, this case demonstrates the power of a gentle process of *shaping* behaviour until it increasingly approximates whatever is desired. It is just like shaping the recalcitrant rat to press the bar. Finally, of course, it was purely behaviour that was dealt with, and to begin with only very simple behaviour in a very simple way. This apparently unim-portant behaviour was gradually built up into fully fledged social be-haviour. Whether at this point in the procedure it would be expedient to continue with this type of therapy is another matter. Certainly, by this stage the patient could be communicated with (at no time in the build-up had he received any instructions) and this would be of benefit to any form of therapy which was pursued thereafter.

Case 2: Stealing, Hoarding and Wearing Excessive Clothes (Ayllon, 1963)

This case also took place in the ward of a mental hospital and involved a 47-year-old female who had been there for nine years, again diagnosed as a schizophrenic. Apart from her other troubles the nursing staff had to spend an enormous amount of time caring for her for three reasons: she stole food, she hoarded the ward's towels in her room, and she wore excessive clothing. The behaviour therapist dealt with these three aspects of her behaviour separately.

(a) Food Stealing. The patient weighed over 250 lb. at the start of the experiment mainly because she ate all the usual food plus whatever she could steal. Persuasion, coaxing and coercion had done nothing to alter this. The therapist assigned her to a table alone in the dining-room. From then onwards whenever she moved towards another table or

attempted to take extra food she was physically removed from the dining-room. In practice, whenever she tried to steal food, she missed an entire meal. Food stealing soon disappeared and her weight dropped to a more respectable level. Like the patient in case study 1, at no time in this procedure was she given any verbal instructions.

(b) Hoarding. Nursing staff had been unable to stop the patient hoarding towels. Instead, roughly twice a week they would go and remove them from her room. Instead of continuing to do this, they were instructed in a straightforward programme of stimulus satiation. From time to time throughout the day a nurse would take a towel and hand it to the patient without comment when she was in her room. In a short period of time the grand total of towels in her room rose to 625, at which point she began to take them out. She did this systematically until there was no more hoarding. A reinforcer loses its power when there is too much of it. In this case the behaviour was changed without ever finding out why the towels had been a reinforcer in the first place; this would have been extremely difficult to do.

(c) Clothing. The patient both wore and carried vast amounts of clothing. To combat this the therapist required her to step onto some scales just before each meal time and meet a particular weight. The limit of the weight requirement was set just below her actual weight plus the weight of the clothes she had worn on the previous day. If she failed the requirement then she missed the meal. After 11 days her clothing weighed 3 lb. rather than the 25 lb. it had weighed to begin with.

These three changes in behaviour led to the patient having more and more social contacts simply because she had become more socially acceptable. This in itself was reinforcing and steady improvement continued. Again throughout this case concentration was on behaviour and how to change it rather than on speculation about deep-seated needs. The actual behaviours were observed and recorded and then specific techniques worked out to deal with each of them.

Case 3: Anorexia (Bachrach, Erwin & Mohr, 1965)

This case was of a female aged 37 who had been diagnosed as anorexic for many years. When the study began she weighed only 47 lb. She could not have been thinner and remained alive. She had many ulcers on her body, had broken numerous bones, presumably through muscular weakness, and could stand only with assistance.

Looked at behaviourally, the problem with anorexia nervosa is that one of the primary reinforcers – food – seems to have lost all its reinforcing power. Search must therefore be made for some other reinforcer which does have some efficacy. For treatment the patient was removed from her pleasant room to one which was barren except for the minimum of amenities. The cooperation of all staff and visitors (which she was temporarily not allowed to receive) was obtained. She was given no further drugs, no psychotherapy and was allowed no conversations and no entertainment. Each of the three experimenters took one meal per day with the patient and used what might be called a gross schedule of reinforcement; this involved the verbal reinforcement of any movement to do with eating. For example, if the patient lifted her fork apparently in the direction of spearing some food then the person eating with her would immediately start to talk of some interesting topic. In this way she was gradually shaped to successive approximations to eating.

Having achieved this much the experimenters made the amount the patient ate determine the post-prandial reinforcement she received. Thus with more food consumed she was allowed more time with the television, record-player, radio, etc. – each of which provided stimuli which were reinforcing to her. If she did not eat, then she received no such reinforcement, a regime which was strictly kept to. The patient reached a new plateau of weight at 63 lb. after which reinforcement was made contingent upon weight gain rather than on amount consumed. In this way her weight was gradually built up again.

When her weight had reached an acceptable level, the patient was started on a course of outpatient treatment which was aimed at getting her new eating behaviour to generalise. Her family's co-operation was achieved in: avoiding any reinforcement of invalid behaviour, not making an issue of eating, reinforcing weight increases verbally, discussing only pleasant topics at meal times, never allowing her to eat alone, setting a rigid schedule for meals, always having one distinctive table-cloth (as a discriminative stimulus for eating), and encouraging her to dine out under enjoyable conditions. These strictures led to a continued gain in weight and an expansion of social activities. The patient eventually retrained successfully and entered the nursing profession to follow a new career.

These three case studies give the flavour of the very different and sometimes quite extreme disorders which can be dealt with by the many techniques of behaviour modification. Whatever form such techniques take they always reflect one set of guiding principles: a constant return to an analysis of what is wrong sheerly in terms of behaviour, what maintains this behaviour and how the environment can be manipulated to change it.

There are countless examples of the application of these principles in the much simpler problems of everyday life. For instance, if a child throws temper tantrums these will eventually stop if they are totally and remorselessly ignored. They will extinguish, although in the early stages of so doing the parents have to put up with much noise and even more heart-ache. Of course, in establishing this type of control it helps if the causes of the behaviour can be found. But this is often difficult, if not impossible. The strength of behaviour modification is that although finding causes is helpful, it is not absolutely necessary in affecting changes in the behaviour.

The Behaviour Therapist

At this point it is worth saying a few words about the behaviour therapist, since he does have characteristics which distinguish him from other therapists, and because of this he is sometimes criticised. His major defining characteristics are a very clear-cut orientation towards theories and principles of learning and an interest in precise behavioural definitions of mental disorders, rather than in speculations about the internal dynamics of the abnormal condition.

In criticism of this approach it is sometimes said that the behaviour therapist is not interested in people, but is merely concerned with their behaviour. Such a criticism is based on the assumption that 'people' can be separated from their behaviour and that this behaviour is a superficial covering over the 'real' person within. Although this is a very commonly held assumption it is not one which the behaviour therapist can make. Instead he assumes that it is impossible to distinguish between a person and his behaviour; a person *is* his behaviour. Of course, it is impossible to say whether or not an assumption is correct since it is little more than an article of faith. It is however worth thinking around this problem in order to have an opinion about which of the two assumptions might lead to the more fruitful approach to therapy.

The other major criticism which is levelled at the behaviour therapist is that he is cold, dictatorial and undemocratic; in other words, that he plays God. This criticism is made because he typically manipulates the environment in a systematic and rather remorseless response-contingent manner in order to change behaviour. When put like this, his behaviour does smack of a 'big brother' attitude with a taint of indoctrination about it.

If it is expanded a little, this criticism opens up a strange dilemma.

Traditional psychotherapy itself has very similar aims to those of behaviour modification, as does the bringing up of children; namely, to help people solve what have been traditionally termed their 'mental' problems and to play a normal part in society. So it is just as manipulative, and hints just as much at indoctrination and the like, as does behaviour modification. But the aims of psychotherapy and of controlling people in everyday life are not expressed as forthrightly as those of behaviour modification, neither are they as obviously manipulative. Also the alternatives to behaviour therapy are couched in terms of the medical model, and at least in some instances they do not work as well as behaviour therapy. It is probably for this reason above all others that people prefer not to have much to do with behaviour modification. Naturally enough perhaps people seem not to mind their behaviour being changed when it is not done so obviously and systematically as it is by the behaviour modifier.

Some of the problems mentioned in this section involve the making of value judgements and moral decisions. There are no definite answers to these and it is best that you draw your own conclusions about them.

Self-Control

It has been clearly established that in many instances behaviour modification is effective; in some ways it can almost be seen as a very practical implementation of common sense. Whether it is more or less effective than other forms of therapy is difficult to determine and perhaps does not matter a great deal given that it is sometimes effective. However, two important questions remain: how can a person be made *less susceptible* to the future development of maladaptive behaviour? and can a person be taught to eliminate such behaviour *without* the aid of the therapist? Eventually the aim must be to enable the patient to be his own therapist, to modify his own behaviour. This is how the behaviour modifer would define self-control.

Speaking non-behaviourally, self-control concerns volition, inner-direction and will-power. Behaviourally it can be characterised simply as using one response to control another response. Good self-control would be achieved if a person could make some responses that effectively inhibit other, undesirable or injurious responses. Probably the best known everyday example of this comes from slimming. Food is taken less frequently and in smaller quantities to prevent the person from over-eating, all being controlled by the very aversive thought of obesity. A number of behavioural techniques have been used as devices of self-control. However, these have mainly taken one of two forms —

reciprocal inhibition and operant control.

Reciprocal Inhibition – Classical Conditioning

(1) As mentioned previously, *relaxation* has been used extensively as a part of desensitisation. However, it has also been seen as a useful self-control technique by teaching a person how to relax at home as well as in therapy. Typically, the person learns to repeat the word 'relax' whenever he begins to relax. In this way, the word eventually stands as a discriminative stimulus for relaxation, the person reducing tension simply by saying the word.

(2) *Desensitisation* has been used in self-control in much the same way as it has in ordinary therapy. However, in this case the person presents the previously constructed hierarchy of anxiety-producing stimuli to himself, whilst initiating self-controlled relaxation.

(3) *Covert sensitisation* is based on aversion therapy – the association of unpleasant, aversive stimuli with undesired behaviour. Here, the idea is to prevent maladaptive behaviours such as stealing, drinking, or smoking by preceding them with *imagined* noxious stimuli. Naturally, before attempting this the therapist has to explain carefully the ideas and implications on which it is based.

For example, the person might be instructed to imagine smoking whilst also imagining that he not only feels sick but is also vomiting luridly and horribly. Then he imagines abstaining from smoking and hence feeling relief from the sickness.

Clearly, covert sensitisation involves a two stage process. (a) In the imagination aversive stimuli are made to follow whatever response is to be reduced – smoking, in the example above. (b) The patient is instructed in ways of imagining escape from the unpleasantness. Those investigators who have worked with this self-control technique (e.g. Cautella, 1967) say that it is successful and that the patients finally report that they no longer feel the need for the particular stimulus. Although such successes have been observed, one question remains unanswered: how does the therapist motivate the individual to sit and quietly destroy with his imagination what is obviously an important reinforcing stimulus in his life? At present such techniques would seem to require the co-operation of a patient who 'wants' to give up the maladaptive behaviour – to kick the habit.

Operant Control – Instrumental Conditioning

The basic assumption of this approach to self-control is that the behaviour an individual *desires* in himself can be achieved with the same methods that would be used to control another person's behaviour. Any of the specific techniques begin with a functional analysis of behaviour much as that made in this chapter and the last, and then the patient and the therapist work together to design individual strategies of learning. There are many such strategies, the following three merely providing examples.

(1) New behaviour. The obvious example of using operant techniques comes from combining novel stimuli with new contingencies of reinforcement to produce new learning; a straightforward attempt to alter the conditions in which maladaptive behaviour occurs. Via instruction from the therapist the old undesirable behaviour is changed by changing the conditions which bring it about.

For example, a married couple who seem unable to stop quarrelling are instructed to make a complete re-arrangement of their household rooms, decor and furniture. They remove all the old discriminative stimuli which have set the scene for bickering, and allow the new stimuli to occasion new responses. Or an even more obvious example comes from the effective way in which over-eating can be controlled by the person simply making food less accessible; by having less of it in the house and by making sure that what there is is not easily accessible — cakes on very high shelves rather than in low cupboards for instance.

(2) Progressive narrowing. Some maladaptive behaviours are difficult to deal with because not only do they lead to immediate positive reinforcement, but they occur very frequently and in a wide variety of situations. They have many discriminative stimuli to promote them. Such behaviours can be brought under self-control by a progressive narrowing of the stimulus control which sets them up. Again, dealing with marital quarrelling, Goldiamond was faced with a husband who often sulked. He instructed him to sulk only on a special (sulking) stool which was always kept in a particular place. He could sulk at any time but *only* on the stool. The sulking soon disappeared.

(3) Immediate support. It is possible to reinforce oneself in order to provide an immediate support for some new behaviour as a sort of temporary measure until the long-term goals are apparent. For example, a person who cannot concentrate on studying for examinations would benefit from breaking up the day into relatively short bursts of study interlaced with many recreational breaks (for coffee, reading novels, or whatever he finds pleasant). The reinforcers would be set up in such a

way that they would be made contingent on set amounts of study.

Assessment of Self-control

By now there is ample evidence that self-control works and that when it does it enjoys some advantages over other forms of therapy. To a large extent a patient's privacy is maintained since there is little in the way of direct observation and manipulation by the therapist. The therapist does not have to obtrude very much into the patient's private life. Therefore, self-control techniques are particularly useful for behaviours which are very private (such as sex) or very frequent (such as eating or smoking).

Secondly, if it can be demonstrated to a person that he has established effective self-control this will probably tend to increase his self-esteem and self-confidence, which in turn should help him to establish even more self-control. For once a vicious circle is set up which is a help rather than a hindrance. When a person has grasped the idea that his behaviour is linked to environmental stimuli then he can begin to arrange his own environment. Some psychologists even believe that new learned behaviour is more likely to be kept up if the person believes that he has been responsible for it himself. Although seductive, this idea still needs to be verified.

On the negative side, self-control has some disadvantages in comparison with other forms of therapy. It can only be used by patients who are in a position to make reliable self-observations and self-reports. Also such techniques can be misused and hence make matters worse. So the person must fully understand at least some of the principles of behaviour modification and be willing to try to apply them. Finally, and perhaps most important, the person must live in an environment in which there exist the necessary reinforcers and stimuli and in which there are places and opportunities for practice. Since these conditions almost certainly involve the co-operation of other people in the person's life, they are by no means always easy to obtain.

Conclusions

The modification of maladaptive behaviour demonstrates some of the ways in which it is possible and useful to apply laboratory derived principles of simple conditioning and learning, although there are many other such examples which come from everyday learning. It remains to say a little about the advantages of these techniques, be they carried out by the therapist directly or by the person's exercise of self-control.

In this context, any classification of maladaptive responses or mental disorder is based on an individual's *current behaviour* and on the stimuli in his environment which bring it about, maintain it, and which might be potentially usable in altering it. It does not therefore involve the difficult and sometimes impossible search through past history for conceivable causes, nor does it involve any awkward analysis of mental or internal states. It is therefore applicable across cultures and sub-cultures, since it is concerned with a direct description of specific behaviour and related aspects of the environment. Although the behaviours which are thought maladaptive might vary from place to place and time to time, this does not matter since the behaviour modifier simply observes, records and manipulates, rather than making any value judgements — at least in his professional capacity.

Overall, behaviour modification is very explicit and is based on a sound knowledge of some of the principles by which new behaviour is learned, conditioned, maintained, strengthened or weakened. This means that much can be done towards altering a repertoire of behaviours that are regarded as deficient, inappropriate or maladaptive, and that are of little value to the individual or to his family and friends, or to society at large.

Summary Points

(1) Behaviour modification is concerned with the application of the principles of conditioning to the alteration of maladaptive behaviour, and exemplifies some of the many ways in which these principles have been usefully applied.

(2) In focusing on behaviour the psychologist involved casts aside the traditional medical model of mental disorder or disease, preferring to conceive of such disorders as learned habits which are deemed maladaptive by the individual or by society.

(3) Ways in which 'bad' habits are learned closely parallel those in which 'good' habits are learned.

(4) There are many ways of modifying behaviour, some based on classical conditioning, others on instrumental conditioning. Whatever form they take however, they all involve the systematic use of stimuli in the environment to alter a person's responses.

(5) Behaviour modifiers have made an interesting analysis of self-control which many psychologists would believe to be the ideal aim of behavioural control. Again, techniques based on classical and instrumental conditioning have been devised for a person to use in controlling his own behaviour. Although useful, such techniques depend very much on

the willingness of the patient to use them in an environment in which this is possible.

(6) The comparative effectiveness of behaviour modification with respect to other types of therapy remains to be properly assessed, although it has been clearly proven effective in many instances. In spite of this there is often great resistance to it, perhaps because of its very explicit aims and methods.

Study Questions – 3

(1) What might be the advantages and disadvantages of regarding mental disease as learned maladaptive habits? To what extent do you think that such habits come into *any* illness?

(2) Give examples of any mild forms of abnormal behaviour that you have seen in general hospitals. What makes them abnormal? What is there in the hospital environment that maintains them?

(3) To what extent do you think that the techniques of behaviour modification might be relevant to general medicine? How might medical practitioners benefit from a knowledge of such techniques?

(4) Discuss some of the ways in which you habitually use behaviour modification principles in your contact with patients and with other people in the paramedical professions.

(5) It can be argued that the ultimate aim of any type of therapy is to enable a patient to achieve self-control. Does this apply equally well to your ultimate aims in dealing with patients?

(6) Outline a programme of self-control techniques that would enable a patient to: lose weight; stop biting his nails; be less hypochondriac.

(7) To what extent is the effect that we all have on one another in our everyday lives and jobs just a rather haphazard form of behaviour modification?

(8) Do you think that all the people you deal with professionally would be equally susceptible to the techniques of behaviour modification? If not, what brings about the differences between them and what is significant about those people whose behaviour you think it would be hard to modify?

(9) How might you attempt to exercise self-control techniques to modify your own behaviour with respect to your patients and your colleagues?

(10) Using principles of conditioning and learning, and the techniques of behaviour modification, broadly applied, do you think that it would be possible to train anyone to become a successful member of one of

the caring professions? If so, how would you change the present system of training along such lines? If not, why would some people be untrainable?

4 THE MANAGEMENT OF LEARNING

The previous two chapters have dealt with conditioning, both in the laboratory and in some applied settings. Conditioning, be it classical or instrumental, is often referred to as *simple* learning. This is not a derogatory term, but one which serves to distinguish it from other types of learning in which psychologists have generally taken a broader view of what is occurring. This is learning as it is more commonly thought of; for example, the learning of new skills, such as driving or typing or playing tennis, or the type of learning that children do in schools, ranging from the words of a carol to Pythagoras's theorem.

This is not the place to consider in any detail whether or not the principles of conditioning are sufficient to account for these broader, more molar types of learning. Psychologists tend to be rather divided on this question. However, although conditioning is relevant to the learning of skills, so are other matters which would rarely be taken into consideration in studies of conditioning. It is with these phenomena that the present chapter is concerned.

The first source of influence on large scale learning, and one with which it is important to deal in these introductory remarks, is *motivation*. As will be apparent by reference to Chapter 9, motivation affects any learning, although it is sometimes difficult to say exactly how and to decide how to measure the strength of the effect. The two points which will now be made about motivation serve as a bridge between this chapter and the two previous chapters.

The first point concerns the motivational role of positive reinforcement when it is used in a broad learning context, rather than in a Skinner box. For example, in one study (Hall, Lund & Jackson, 1968), the investigators asked teachers to point out which were the most disruptive children in their classrooms. Then for some weeks ratings were taken of the work habits of these children. In the manipulative part of the study, an observer in the classroom would hold up a coloured card when a particular (disruptive) child was working normally; it could be seen only by the teacher. The teacher would then go up to the child and praise him. (With disruptive children, the common response is to pay them attention only when they are being disruptive, and not when they are not.)

This procedure had the effect of pushing up study time from 25 per cent to between 60 per cent and 90 per cent in individual cases. When the reinforcement was discontinued, study time decreased, and then rose again when it was reinstituted. The overall result was a general improvement in academic performance.

Here then is an example of an obviously external or extrinsic reinforcer acting as a motivator of rather broad aspects of study and learning. In the real world, most sources of motivation do seem to be extrinsic, taking the form of badges, stars, money, praise, medals, and so on. These are all stimuli which have nothing directly to do with whatever activity they are promoting. However, it is generally thought that learning proceeds more effectively if the motivation comes more intrinsically; i.e. is a more inevitable corollary of the activity itself. Although this extrinsic/intrinsic distinction is sometimes a little arbitrary, it is possible to think of fairly clear examples of intrinsic motivation. For instance, learning to write carries with it the obvious benefits of being better able to express ideas. Learning to walk or to ride a bicycle carry the obvious advantages of being better able to move around the environment.

More extremely, it would seem that learning can sometimes be its *own reward* and be engaged in simply for its own sake. Learning involves curiosity and exploration which do seem to be innately important, at least to some people. It follows from this discussion that in practical terms it is important for a teacher to find ways of making whatever is being learned have its intrinsic benefits and to exploit these. One way in which this idea has been explored in schools is to make the doing of more desired intellectual activities dependent on some period of time spent on less favoured intellectual pursuits. In this way intrinsic benefits are being built into the general system of teaching and learning.

Apart from their more obvious advantages, intrinsic rewards meet two objections which can otherwise be levelled against the use of extrinsic rewards. A planned external reward is rather like a bribe and may lead whoever receives it to learn to be docile and deferent to the authority which hands it out, rather than to be spontaneous and creative. Also, most extrinsic rewards are competitive, so some learners will always be doomed to failure. Whether or not this is judged to be a bad state of affairs will, of course, depend on what alternative sources of benefit are made available to those who fail.

These general points about motivation should be borne in mind throughout the remainder of this chapter since they are constantly relevant to any of the more molar types of learning. Also relevant are phenomena such as thinking, and problem solving, remembering and forgetting. However, these topics are so important in their own right (as of course is motivation) that they have been accorded individual chapters and will not be pursued further in this one.

Skills

Skills are defined as organised *patterns* of responses. Although it is conceivable that they can be broken down into relatively discrete facets, to the learning of each of which the principles of conditioning might be relevant, they still have to be learned in a total, organised sense. It is in this respect that other influences make themselves felt.

Arguably, the most general characteristics of the learning of skills is that the rate at which it occurs tends to be similar from one skill to the next, even though the precise time sequences involved might differ. To take typing for example, there is a rapid improvement (faster performance and fewer errors) throughout the first 15 or 20 hours of learning. Thereafter, the rate of improvement slows down until there are many hours in which there appears to be no improvement at all. Such flat parts in the learning curve are known as *plateaux*. Eventually, however, the rate of learning increases again until a new plateau is reached. This usually means that some new level of the skill has become organised. In typing this might mean that the person has now learned to type in flowing word sequences rather than in letter sequences, for example.

Although such improvements in performance interspersed with plateaux are typical of the rate at which skills are learned, there is a problem of interpretation. If one plots a curve of learning against time, inevitably one is taking a measure of *performance*, and making inferences from this about learning. It is impossible to measure the learning directly. Of course, conditions other than learning will affect performance; for example, local transient changes in mood, emotional state, motivation etc. It is therefore important to be careful in deciding whether any changes in the rate at which a skill is being performed or in the number of errors which are being made are due to temporary conditions or are the reflections of permanent learning.

Massed Versus Distributed Practice

One of the most important variables that affects the learning of skills is the way in which the practice is arranged. Imagine that you have a day in which to learn the rudiments of a skill such as typing or driving; do you concentrate all your efforts into continuous practice or do you distribute your practice and intersperse it with periods of rest? The broad answer to this question is that distributed practice leads to more effective learning of sensorimotor skills, i.e. those that require eye-hand co-ordination for example, than does massed practice. On the other hand, massed practice is often more effective when the task involves a great deal of thought. In general, the advantages of distributed practice lessen as tasks become more complex.

There are a number of theories to account for the relative advantages of distributed and massed practice, although which of them will be best supported remains to be seen. For example, one view rests on an analysis of whether or not a person's tendencies to make errors are extinguished. The argument is that all the potential errors that a person brings to the learning situation with him will extinguish more easily when practice is distributed than massed, and that this will produce more effective learning.

An alternative view is that of *consolidation* theory which assumes that the full effect of whatever underlies learning takes some time to occur and the leaving of gaps between practice allows this 'setting' process to happen without interference. One way in which this argument has been extended is to say that if interference of other things hinders consolidation, then material learned just before sleep should be better retained than that learned just before waking activity. In general this seems to be so, however again only with the more simple forms of task. Overall, the best arrangement for practice in the learning of skills seems to be frequent bursts of activity interpolated with short periods of rest.

Parts Versus Wholes

If a person has a long and complicated task or skill to learn is it better to tackle the task as a whole or to break it down into parts? The early studies which bore on this question produced results which favoured the whole method, whereas some later studies were somewhat ambiguous in their findings. As is often the case in psychology a seemingly simple and harmless question has to be answered in a complex way.

McGeoch and Iron (1952) summarised the factors which have to be taken into account in the part/whole problem. Although this summary was made such a relatively long time ago, it still stands. It is best expressed as a series of points.

(1) A more *intelligent* learner can use the whole method more advantageously than one who is less intelligent. Of course, in the context of the learning of skills 'more' and 'less' will depend on some of the points below.

(2) The advantages of the whole method increase with *practice.*

(3) If practice is *distributed* then the whole method is advantageous.

(4) The whole method outweighs the part method if the material to be learned is *meaningful,* continuous prose rather than jumbled lists of words for example.

(5) The total *length* of the task and its numbers of obvious parts are relevant. For example, if a task happens to divide in very straightforward ways then it would be best so to divide it.

(6) The relative disadvantage of the whole method comes from the time which is necessary to *connect the parts* once they have been learned.

From these points it is fair to say that with long tasks the whole method is generally to be preferred over the part method. However, a further factor needs to be taken into account. In learning complex material there is what is called a *serial position effect.* This simply describes the fact that the beginning and end of the material is learned more readily than the middle sections. If the whole method were being followed then the beginning and end would be overlearned in order to ensure that the middle was learned to a reasonable standard. This might be the case when learning a poem for example. If the serial position effect is at work then part learning would seem to be advisable, at least to the extent of starting and ending the 'part' just before and just after the more difficult middle material.

Meaningfulness

To introduce a discussion of the effects of meaningfulness on complex learning, it is useful to mention the *nonsense syllable.* This was devised in the last century by Ebbinghaus in an effort to study what he considered to be 'pure' memory, that is, memory which is unhampered and unaffected by a person's knowledge of the items to be remembered. The nonsense syllable is always of three letters, and always in the form consonant-vowel-consonant, e.g. WUJ; also, it is not a recognised word in the language. Although Ebbinghaus believed that such syllables had no meaning, this is not quite the case in that they have since been shown to have various *association values.* Thus, for example, most people would produce more associations to HAV than to QIJ. Nevertheless, all nonsense syallables can be graded as to their association value (and hence their meaning) and thus provide one way of comparing the learning of meaningful material with the learning of that which is *relatively* meaningless.

As might be expected, the general relationship between learning and meaning is that the more meaningful items happen to be, the more readily they are learned. For example, random lists of meaningful words are learned more easily than random lists of nonsense syllables which are highly suggestive of words. In their turn, the latter are learned faster and with fewer errors than are the less suggestive nonsense syllables.

In a similar way, material which is patterned or organised is more readily learned than material which is not. For example, intelligible prose is learned more effectively than are lists of random words, and by a similar token, poetry (with its greater patterning and more obvious structure — usually) is learned faster than prose of the same length.

To take the idea of meaning up one level, it is important to consider the effect of what might be called understanding on learning, particularly when dealing with written material. In this regard, the memory for the basic ideas of a passage which a person says that he understands is retained more permanently than the same passage learned by rote. Although retention is more directly concerned with memory than with original learning, the two phenomena are related.

An addendum to the effect of meaning on learning is *feedback* or *knowledge of results*. When a person is learning something, on occasion he is given feedback as to how he is progressing, whether he is right or wrong, and on occasion, not. The learning of skills and complex tasks proceeds more readily if knowledge of results is given along the way. Without feedback it is impossible to be accurate. Some would say that even a rat in a Skinner box has feedback, in the way of reinforcement. And in practice it is very difficult to separate the effects on learning of the reward given by a reinforcing stimulus from its informational or feedback properties. In general, immediate feedback is more efficacious than delayed feedback and learning progresses more readily if the person is also given information about the size and direction of any errors he might make.

Activity Versus Passivity

When approaching the learning of a new task it is possible to spend all one's time reading or looking or in some similar activity; or, alternatively one can spend a proportion of the available time in rehearsing the material. In general, it has been found that with verbal material and rote learning, it is best if some 20 per cent of the time is spent reading and 80 per cent spent rehearsing. Also, vocalisation of the material aids learning, as in fact does *doing* anything that might be involved. Learning is more effective when active rather than passive.

On the basis of research carried out into active versus passive learning, Voeks (1964) offers some interesting advice to college students, which is, of course, relevant to anyone who is pursuing the complex learning involved in higher education generally.

(1) When learning avoid too much in the way of relaxation. In other words, do not sit too comfortably and relaxed; keep muscles reasonably tense.

(2) Immediately after a class has finished review the material which has been covered in it.

(3) When reading, be active rather than passive. That is, think about what is being read rather than just letting it flow in whilst perhaps thinking vaguely of other things.

(4) Read with the goal of answering questions about the material.

(5) Do not just memorise any material to be learned, but also think about its implications and ways in which it might generalise.

(6) Practise asking intelligent questions derived from the material being learned.

(7) Take abundant notes.

(8) Record questions when they suggest themselves rather than leaving them until later.

(9) Be active, attentive and responsive in class.

(10) When studying for examinations, ask and answer questions.

(11) If certain details have to be remembered, then recite them.

In general, of course, Voeks is saying that to be successful the learner of complex material is better off being active rather than passive in every way that he can think of.

Transfer of Training

Against the cry of 'What are we doing this for?' some schoolmasters used to justify the study of Latin on the grounds that it trained the mind. This was a reflection of the idea that the mind is a mixture of faculties which can be strengthened through exercise; a curious picture of the mental being physically quantifiable. Such ideas have been totally discredited; Latin does not train the mind. However, training or learning can be transferred in other ways, both positively (to enhance learning) and negatively (to impede learning).

There are two ways in which transfer of training is thought to occur. The first is known as *transfer through similarity*. The idea here is that when two sets of material to be learned have very similar components, then the second will be learned more easily than the first. A person learning new material takes advantage of whatever it might have in common with earlier experiences and thereby eases the new learning a little.

There are many examples of transfer through similarity, both verbal and non-verbal. For instance, there is one way in which learning Latin does aid future learning. An integral part of the learning of Latin is to come to terms with its grammatical structure. To have done this makes the grammatical structure of English easier to understand and learn. To take a more practical example, the transfer of learning through similarity is often employed in the teaching of skills such as driving or flying by using simulators. In this case, the controls and general conditions are identical from the simulated situation to the real one, except, of course, for the person's knowledge that he is in a simulator.

A special case of transfer of training is found with *paired associate* learning. This is a technique which is very commonly used to study verbal learning in the laboratory. Items to be learned are arranged in pairs and the subject works through a list, being shown the first item of each pair with the instruction to respond by giving the second item. The presentation of successive lists of paired associates offers a good opportunity to study transfer of training. It has been found that a second list is learned with more facility if the stimulus words are similar between the two lists and the response words are the same. On the other hand, there is *negative* transfer if the stimulus words are the same between the two lists but the response words are different. The learning of the second list is worse than it would have been had the first list not been learned.

The second type of transfer is termed *transfer through principles*. Put another way, this refers to learning to learn. It is the use of a previously learned principle in a new application. Although this often has a positive effect on learning there are some cases in which it does not. It is important to bear in mind transfer through principles when teaching. For example, in academic terms, the principles of reasoning which are learned as a part of mathematics can be applied with benefit to the learning of logic.

A special (and useful) case of this type of learning is known as *bilateral* transfer, which refers to transfer of something learned on one side of the body to the other side. For example, if you cover a person's hand so that he can only see it in a mirror and then get him to trace round an awkwardly shaped drawing, he will find great difficulty in this. Then let him practise the task with the other hand until he has mastered the principles of it, and you will find that he can do it immediately with the first hand. A useful principle.

Sometimes, however, transfer through principles can lead to negative outcomes. A good example of this comes in learning racket sports which, of course, share a similarity of equipment. However, the principles of good stroke play in tennis are very different from those in squash or badminton. This means that in the initial stages of learning there may well be negative transfer from one sport to the other. For example, it would be very poor play in tennis to use the wrist as much as it would be used in squash.

Overall, the results of the study of transfer of training can be summarised quite briefly. Transfer of training occurs but it is very much *less* than might be expected. The amount of transfer depends partially on the method of teaching and hence on the method of learning. Fortunately, good habits of study appear to transfer easily, although transfer is not automatic even when the possibilities exist for it.

Teaching Machines and Programmed Learning

Many of the principles of complex learning described above have been put together with those of instrumental conditioning in research which has gone into the development of teaching machines and the programmed learning which they make possible. Essentially a student can work at his own pace when using a teaching machine. Typically, he is faced with a small machine in which there is a slot through which he reads a question. He selects what he believes to be the correct answer to this and presses a corresponding button. If he is right the next question drops into the slot and he proceeds. If he is wrong then a different statement or question is presented and he carries on from there. Naturally, at each question there are usually a number of choices, any errors that are made leading to different outcomes in the progression of the learning.

As might be expected, the force of teaching machines depends on the thought and creativity which goes into their programming. Since the material itself is intended to do the teaching, it is crucial that it be arranged in a form in which it can be most easily mastered. The general principle which determines this is that of presenting information and then letting the learner participate by supplying answers that have already been hinted at or prompted. There is a constant interchange between the learner and the material.

There are various ways in which responses are prompted. For example, there might be similarity of ideas: 'Just as letters arranged into words are learned more readily than jumbled letters, so organised word sequences are ——— ——— ——— than jumbled word sequences.' Or there might be grammatical restrictions: 'Stimuli and responses are connected by associations. So the learner associates 10 with 5 x 2 or he ———graphite and wood cylinders with pencils.'

The considerable success enjoyed by teaching machines and pro-grammed instruction (which can occur in book form, without the teaching machine) particularly with factual material, illustrates three main points.

(1) The learner is very *active*, responding, practising and testing at each step in his process of learning.

(2) The learner finds out with the *minimum of delay* whether or not his response is *correct*; he gains immediate feedback and/or reinforcement.

(3) The learner can move ahead on an individual basis entirely at his own rate, thereby reducing the difficulties of teaching a group of students of very mixed abilities.

Although there has been a great deal of research into the efficacy of teaching machines, there remain some unanswered questions. For example, when asking a question, is it better to require a short answer or a response to a multiple choice? For instance, either: 'A stimulus-response association is strengthened through ————?' (Reinforcement) Or: 'A stimulus-response association is strengthened through: (a) extinc-tion, (b) *reinforcement*, (c) discrimination, (d) generalisation.' Also, should the student have to be so active as to write the answer, or can he just think it? How large should the steps be in the learning process? And so on.

There are two obvious disadvantages of teaching machines. First, if the material is very complex and highly theoretical it is very difficult to programme. So, although it might be reasonable to write a programme for introductory anatomy, it would be more problematical with philo-sophy. Second, and more important, interaction between the learner and the teacher is reduced and the learning situation is by that much at least potentially less flexible. However, the use of teaching machines has added to the knowledge of how people learn and has suggested for example that individual differences between normally slow and nor-mally fast learners are reduced when this method is used.

Conclusions

The study of how complex skills are acquired and difficult material is learned highlights principles of a quite different order from those seen in classical and instrumental conditioning. These principles devolve from the motivational state of the learner, from the nature of the material itself, and from the manner of learning. They are put into prac-tice in the construction of teaching machines and in the way in which these are programmed.

Summary Points

(1) Broad aspects of motivation affect the way in which complex material is learned. Of particular importance is the effect of praise (positive reinforcement) and whether the motivation is extrinsic or intrinsic. In general, intrinsic motivation promotes more effective learning.

(2) Typically, the rate at which complex skills are learned conforms to a pattern of bursts of improvement followed by flat periods. The main influences on such learning are whether it is done in a massed or distributed way, whether the material is learned as a whole or in parts, the meaningfulness of the material, whether or not feedback is given, and whether the learning is active or passive.

(3) A specific aspect of more broadly based learning is transfer of training from one task to another. This can be positive or negative and can occur through similarity in the material itself or through principles emerging which are common to both tasks.

(4) Principles of complex learning, together with those of conditioning, have been successfully applied to teaching through machines. The efficacy of teaching machines depends very much on the way in which the material for them is programmed, but they have the general advantage of allowing a student to proceed at his own pace.

Study Questions – 4

(1) How would you motivate a patient to learn a new skill or to relearn an old one if he had already expressed a lack of interest in it?

(2) If someone was learning to walk again or to write again after having a stroke, would he improve faster if he were being paid for his progress than if not? How important would be your encouragement of his progress?

(3) Choose some of the tasks that your patients have to cope with, and use these to test the principles which influence the type of learning described in this chapter. That is: test the rate at which new learning occurs, test the effects of different types of practice, test whole versus part learning, test the effects of meaningfulness and feedback, and test the effects of active versus passive roles adopted by the learner.

(4) How would you train someone to write with his other hand? (Compare your answer with that which you gave in the study questions in the second chapter.)

(5) Describe some of the ways in which you already use the principles behind the management of learning in your professional capacity. Are they more appropriate to some people and some situations than to

others?

(6) List ten examples of transfer of training as you have observed them in your own professional training and in your contact with patients. In each case say whether the transfer is positive or negative.

(7) Of yourself and an equally intelligent contemporary why should one do better in training than the other? Of two patients with the same problems and the same basic physical capacities following an accident, why should one return to a normal independent life sooner than the other?

(8) Take any one of the skills you have to learn as part of your training and on the basis of the principles described in this chapter design a series of questions by which it might be taught in a programmed text.

(9) Do you think it possible that the learning of complex skills that sometimes has to be achieved by hospitalised patients might be explicable in terms of conditioning? If so, how? If not, why not?

(10) Would Voeks' advice to students be sufficient to make you do well in your professional studies? Would it help patients to learn new skills and to relearn old ones?

5 MEMORY AND FORGETTING

The major point of this chapter is to turn to the face of the coin which was not shown in the last three chapters on learning. Learning cannot occur without memory and the very human capacity for flexibility could not be displayed without memory. However, as with many other psychological concepts, memory is a hypothetical process. It is obvious that any organism which learns must have memory; but although apparently obvious this is still only an inference. We infer that a person has a memory because he does not constantly have to relearn all that he does, be it driving a car or doing quadratic equations. It might even be said that it would be impossible for him to learn at all without a memory. But all this is only inference; at present psychologists and physiologists cannot point to something in the brain and say that this is memory or that memory is here, although of course it may be that this is possible in the future. So, as with learning and motivation, an understanding of memory comes indirectly through measures of changes in what a person does from time to time.

There are many phenomena which seem to affect memory. For example, interest, motivation and knowledge all have an influence. Consider two persons walking through a town for the first time; one is an architect, the other a novelist. After their walk, the architect would have no trouble in remembering what and where the significant buildings were, and the novelist would probably have little trouble in reviewing the appearances and characteristics of the various people they had passed. In all probability, neither would remember much of what was important to the other. It was in order to try to control these complex influences on memory, that so much use has been made of relatively neutral material such as nonsense syllables. Except perhaps to a linguist, it can be assumed that these are no more important or interesting to one person than to the next.

These rather complex matters lead to an immediate array of questions which psychologists (and others) have asked about memory. How does memory work? How do we remember things? Is there more than one kind of memory? Why do some people have better memories than others? What makes people forget things? The latter question points to the other side of memory. Naturally, memory and forgetting are inseparable, but they are often dealt with separately, as they will be here. On the one hand, research and theory have been concerned with a search for memory processes, and on the other, there are various theories of forgetting, with their own sets of evidence.

Remembering

Types of Remembering

Essentially, work on remembering is concerned with finding ways of analysing a person's present responses for signs of responses that he had learned earlier. The three main ways which have been devised to do this can be seen as three types of remembering or simply as three ways in which to measure memory.

(1) Recall. This is the most obvious form of memory. It is what happens when you sit down and think over the events of the day, or when you have a job to do which you have not done for some time you reflect on how you did it. To measure recall, all that is required is a means of showing that present performance is different from what it would have been without some residue from the past; for example, that one could not swim the breast stroke without having previously learned to do so. This can be done very easily with *paired associate* methods (see Chapter 4) or by *serial anticipation* in which the items in a list to be learned are shown one by one and the subject has to use each as a stimulus for the next, to anticipate it by saying or writing it. A measure of how many items a person gets correct on the first occasion he makes the attempt after the initial learning is the recall score.

(2) Recognition. Having seen a face or heard a name only once a person very often cannot recall them, but he might well recognise them again. He might be able to pick out the face or name from similar ones. Laboratory studies of this very common and automatic process must be able to distinguish between correct and faulty recognition. With recall, this is easy; the response is either right or wrong, it is remembered or not. With recognition the stimulus might not be recognised or it might be incorrectly recognised. This problem has led to the development of the recognition score. Imagine that a subject is given 25 photographs with which to familiarise himself. These are then mixed with a further 25 from which he has to sort out those he first saw. His recognition score would be:

$$100 \text{ x } \frac{\text{Right minus wrong}}{\text{Total}}$$

Had he been completely correct his score would be 100 per cent, whereas anything less than half right effectively achieves only 0 per cent.

(3) Relearning. Even though something seems to be completely forgotten, i.e. it cannot be recalled or recognised, it may be that if it is learned a second time, the relearning will be faster and have fewer errors than the first learning. For example, if a person at age 40 can recall virtually nothing of the material he had learned for an examination at age 16, he would probably be able to relearn the material more easily than he had learned it originally.

When studied in the laboratory, relearning obviously needs the same material to be learned on two separate occasions, and to the same *criterion*. (This word 'criterion' refers to how well something is learned. For example, if a list of words is to be learned, it can be learned until perfect, or until it is perfect on three consecutive trials, or until there is only one error, and so on. The setting of a criterion is always an arbitrary matter, usually determined by experimental expediency. What is important is that once set, it is adhered to.) So, if the second learning requires fewer trials than the first in order to reach the same criterion, it is assumed that there have been some *savings* from one to the other. The savings score is:

$$100 \text{ x } \frac{\text{original number of trials minus relearning number of trials}}{\text{original number of trials}}$$

From this simple function it can be seen that if the criterion is reached on the first relearning trial there are 100 per cent savings, and when the relearning takes as long as the original learning, there are 0 per cent savings.

It would seem that the processes underlying these three types of memory may well be distinct. Each appears to make a different demand on the individual, although the nature of these demands is not clear. Suffice it to say that it is far easier to relearn something than it is to recognise it, and far easier to recognise it than it is to recall it.

Earlier work

Recent work and ideas on memory will be discussed below; for now it can be summarised by saying that it has been concerned with the processes underlying memory plus the matter of individual differences. By contrast, the earlier studies were conducted in a search for *universals* in memory and in an attempt to study *pure* memory using nonsense syllables and rote methods.

Ebbinghaus's pioneer work has already been mentioned in Chapter 4. As well as carrying out thousands of what must have been very tedious experiments on himself with nonsense syllables, he also invented the savings method as a measure of memory. Of course, in retrospect it is now possible to say that pure memory cannot be studied. Whatever materials are used must have some association value, even the meaningless-seeming nonsense syllable. And such associations will differ from person to person in unpredictable ways.

There is a similar tradition of work involving *paired-associate* learning. The ease of recall of material learned in this way depends on the nature of the items and on whether the learner is familiar with the stimulus items before the experiment or sees them in it for the first time. Problems in learning and memory involving such material also come from interference between words and associations to be learned and associations which already exist for the individual. In general, studies of paired-associates show learning to be a smooth incremental process, very similar to learning in animals. However, in spite of this it is not possible to conclude that the same processes are involved in learning and remembering.

A rather different tradition of studies in memory is exemplified by a series carried out on children by Piaget. He showed five to seven-year-olds' pictures such as in Figure 5.1a and then asked them to draw them from memory. In doing so they would produce drawings such as in Figure 5.1b.

Asked again to draw the same picture from memory, some 30 per cent of the children did somewhat *better* than they had at first. Piaget established that they had not rehearsed the pictures in the meantime and concluded that the improvement must be due to their development and growth and more mature ideas.

This type of finding is a little akin to the *reminiscence* effect in which retention of material is better after a few minutes than it is immediately following the learning. This effect is by no means always seen but it has been recorded often enough to be well established, particularly in the learning of motor skills.

Figure 5.1 Piaget's Experiment

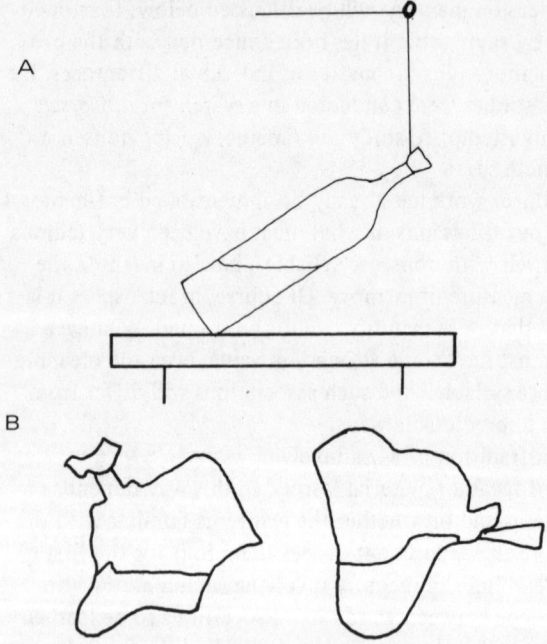

Some investigators have explained effects such as this by suggesting
that they are due to *mental practice*, and there is certainly evidence that
this does aid the learning of motor skills. Be this as it may, effects such
as Piaget's and that of reminiscence weigh against one of the more traditional models of memory. This views memory as a simple storage tank
into which items of stimulus-response associations can be put and from
which they can be retrieved under appropriate conditions. This is a
view of memory as a fairly passive affair. However, although the traditional studies showed rehearsal and rote to be important, they also
point to learning and memory being *active* and selective, and being
affected by a person's interests and abilities.

Sensory Information Storage

Recent work on memory has depended very much on an analysis of
four different processes or concepts. The first of these is sensory information storage, which deals with memory in a very immediate sense, in
fact, with what is happening in the first few *parts of a second* during
which information is incoming. Although this might be thought to be a
difficult area of study an important breakthrough was made by Sperling

(1960). He carried out a series of studies in which he showed subjects sets of stimuli such as:

> 71VF
> XL53
> B4W7

for a few milliseconds (in a tachistoscope). Having seen this type of material for such a brief time, subjects cannot remember it.

Dealing with this very immediate memory, there seems to be a limit of between five and nine items (or the magic number seven, plus or minus two, as it was called by one psychologist). However, Sperling also played three musical tones to his subjects, one high, one medium, and one low. He then showed them the blocks of 12 items for a few milliseconds and immediately sounded one of the tones. Subjects were told that they should regard the tone as corresponding to one of the three lines in the stimulus array — top, middle and bottom. Under these conditions, subjects could recite the items on the relevant line.

At first thought, Sperling's finding may seem trivial, but a little more thought will show that it has important implications. It means that for a *very* short time a person must have an *icon* (a term coined by Neisser, 1966), or a very brief photographic representation, of the stimulus. If he is cued in the right way then he can read off whatever is the appropriate part of the icon, or presumably the whole thing if it is not too complex or does not contain too many items. Such experiments show that this iconic storage of sensory information lasts for about 250 milliseconds. This should be regarded as the very first stage in memory.

Short-term Memory

Under appropriate conditions (of interest, attitude, values, motivation, etc.), material may be encoded and pass from the store of sensory information into short term memory. This next stage of memory is thought usually to last for about 18 seconds. Items do not pass on beyond this stage unless they are actively rehearsed. Think of looking up a telephone number. One can remember it long enough to dial it but will probably have forgotten it a few minutes later unless one has made some active effort to remember it, or unless something has happened to make it stick. On the other hand, if, between looking up the number and dialling it something happens to distract one briefly, one will probably have to look it up again. The information has not passed from short term memory into a more permanent store. (It should be remembered that in these discussions the words 'store' and 'storage' are used in an entirely metaphorical sense. It is useful to think of memories being stored but no one has yet seen such a store directly; it is an analogy.)

Peterson and Peterson (1959) carried out one of the most influential experiments on short term memory. They gave subjects groups of three consonants to learn and then instructed them to start counting backwards in threes from, say, 98. After various times had elapsed they stopped them and asked them to repeat the trigram they had learned. Of course, different subjects were only stopped once for each trigram; they could not be tested repeatedly. It was found that the memory of the trigram disappeared after about 18 seconds of counting.

Although such experiments set fairly precise limits on this stage of memory they left one enormous problem unanswered. Why does the information disappear from memory? Does it just decay with the passing of time or is it interfered with or inhibited by other activity, in this case that which comes from counting backwards in threes? As will be seen later, ideas of decay or interference form the basis of two of the most influential theories of forgetting.

Long-term Memory

As mentioned above, if some positive effort is made, or material is rehearsed, memories appear to become more permanent. Make a conscious effort to rehearse a telephone number and then use it a few times, and one will not only remember it a week later, but will even probably be able to dredge it up in months or years to come. In fact, the problem may be to forget it. This more permanent memory is sometimes known as long term memory, and it should be said at the outset that not a great deal is known about it except at a relatively superficial level. At present, it is not even possible to say whether it is based on neuronal change or electrochemical change, or whatever. However, aspects of it have received serious attention and some of these will be described briefly.

A great deal of speculation has gone into how memory is *organised*, usually in the form of constructing hypothetical models of the processes involved and finding ways of testing them. There is little point here in going into these in detail, except to say that no one of them is generally accepted amongst psychologists, and that the most basic of them is the *storage tank* idea, with memory seen as a fixed, static store. This would seem to be an oversimplified idea since memory appears to be more active than it would imply. Think for example of trying to remember some event from your childhood. This seems to be an active process of recreation and reconstruction. There are many ways in which items can be retrieved from the past, other than just by dipping into a store.

Interestingly, the way in which such memories are organised must have something to do with what is *not* in memory. For example, if someone says a word which is new to you, you know *immediately* that you do not know it. How? This is an amazing process, suggesting that all the words in the private dictionaries of our memories can be scanned at once and the relevant one be judged missing. Try these for example: pica, trichotillomania, echolalia. There is a good chance that you will not know at least one of these and also knew immediately that it was unfamiliar to you.

A second area of study has involved the *form* which memory takes. The basic question here is: how do we record things? Do we record them in memory visually, verbally, or in some other way to which a name cannot be easily given? There is evidence that at least these two, visual and verbal memories exist. Some people are primarily visualisers and others primarily verbalisers. Also, the evidence suggests that visual memory is virtually limitless whereas verbal memory is far more restricted. To decide whether you are mainly a visualiser or a verbaliser, imagine giving instructions to someone about how to travel on a particular route. Do you visualise the route and describe it accordingly or do you remember verbally the sequences of turns and distances? Also, try to remember a long list of items, either verbally or by creating a lurid visual image to go with each. You will find that the latter is far easier.

In recent years, a great deal of attention has been given to *mnemonics*. Of course, people have used such aids to memory for hundreds of years, but have not been much concerned with how they work and what they can tell us of memory. The simplest mnemonics are rhymes (e.g. I before E except after C). It is easy to see that these aid memory by creating a very straightforward organisation. An external constraint is put simultaneously on a great variety of items which would be extremely arduous to remember individually.

The oldest mnemonic device is probably the system of loci, which puts a rather different constraint upon the objects to be remembered. The system simply involves placing the items you want to remember into a series of places that you know very well (a mental exercise of course). You might for example, walk around your house in your imagination putting the items into all the odd corners and cupboards that you know so well. Then, when you wish to remember them, you simply walk round and take them out again. This system works especially well if unusual things are put together, like a matchbox down a plughole, for example.

Another important mnemonic system which works very well is that of *key words*. For example, the digits 1 to 9 might be linked to various objects and then a sequence of digits remembered by odd juxtapositions of the objects. For instance, you might remember a door (4) with a tree (3) through it on which is drawn a line (9) which points to a bun (1). Thus you remember 4391.

Studies of mnemonics indicate that in long term memory organisation is important and that memory is a matter of hard work and not magic. Long term memory is closely linked to *how* the information is acquired in the first place and how it is retrieved. Like the management of learning, memory is an *active* rather than a passive process.

Retrieval

The final process which has engaged the attention of researchers is retrieval. Earlier on, the differences between the various types of retrieval were mentioned — recall, recognition, and relearning. Errors, when they occur in the retrieval process, are of two kinds. There is the obvious error of *omission*, when something is left out. But there are also errors of *commission,* when items are put in which were not there to begin with.

Also important in retrieval is a process known as *confabulation.* For example, motivation affects retrieval. The simplest instance is that people will remember more if they are paid to do so. But if the motivation is very high, then this detracts from retrieval by leading to more errors of commission. Quite simply, people make up (perhaps unconsciously) items to put in, although they might well believe their responses to be genuine.

As was seen with long term memory, the retrieval process depends to some extent on how information is accepted or rejected, how the decision is made. Think for example of when you are trying to remember a name which is on the tip of your tongue. Various possibilities suggest themselves. How do you know whether to reject or to accept them? Is his name Baker or Laker, or Baker or Rolls? The answers to such questions cannot yet be given, but when they can, will tell us much about the process of retrieving memories. It is necessary to know how the information gets in, how it is stored, and how it is drawn out when needed.

Forgetting

There can be no learning without some retention of the material which is taken in. But retention and forgetting present a very paradoxical picture. On the one hand, people seem to retain very little of what they experience; think of how little you can remember of the massive numbers of stimuli which clamour for attention at every waking moment. On the other hand, people seem to remember vast amounts; just think for a moment of *all* the things that you know; within a minute the list becomes enormous. One of the major problems in this rather paradoxical area comes with trying to explain why people forget, particularly when it is frequently to their detriment to do so. Can something which has passed into so-called long term memory be completely forgotten? If so, how and why?

There have been three main approaches to answer such questions, but before describing these it is worth making a few general points about forgetting. The rate of forgetting tends to be as regular as that of learning. If a person is tested for retention at set periods of time after learning then the following function is usually found:

Figure 5.2 Retention Curve

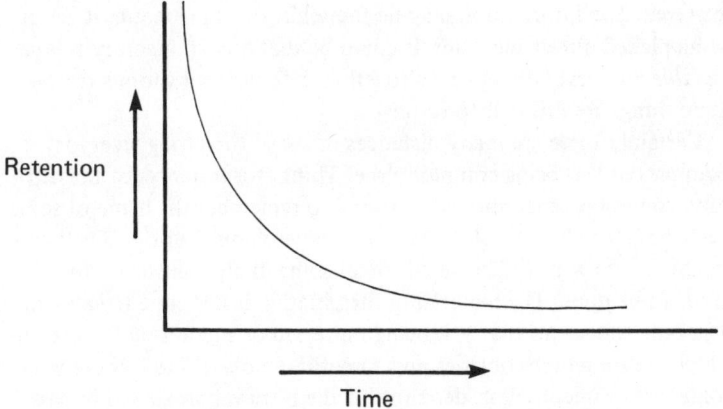

The typical curve falls off rapidly immediately after learning and then tails off gradually. Such curves were established by Ebbinghaus (1913) and have been well endorsed since his time. However, later investigations have shown that the precise rate of forgetting depends on the various materials learned and on the circumstances under which memorising occurs.

In general, motor skills are better retained than verbal materials (perhaps due to mental practice), and meaningful material is better retained than non-meaningful. There is even better and longer retention of information which is gained from solving problems. These effects may be because to learn non-meaningful material the learner has to overcome highly practised habits (such as those of letter and word position) which might well interfere with retention. Such interferences have to be done away with for retention to be improved. It may well be that forgetting is an active process, an idea which is reinforced by work on mnemonics.

The three main explanations of forgetting are: motivated (or intentional) forgetting, decay (or distortion) of the memory trace, and interference (or inhibition) theory. As will be seen below, it is difficult to choose between the appropriateness of these theories and it may be that forgetting is best explained by some *rapprochement* between all three.

Motivated (Intentional) Forgetting

If a memory lasts for a while and then disappears, then acquisition must have worked. But a failure to recall something does not show whether the material is entirely gone from memory or that it is simply not being retrieved. The information may be there but for some reason it is not being picked out of the store. It could be that human memory is *non-erasable* and never disappears altogether, although for various reasons some things are difficult to retrieve.

Certainly there are many instances of social forgetting, everyday examples of this being commonplace. Think, for instance, of the difficulty sometimes encountered in trying to remember the name of someone whom you know well but whom you very much dislike. Or the apparent ease with which we all forget some unpleasant task which needs to be done. The material or information is not gone from memory; rather, it seems that it is being repressed or suppressed for reasons which are sometimes obvious and sometimes not. It is as if there is a conscious or unconscious decision for the retrieval process to bypass the material. This will sometimes even show up in a person's bodily reactions, with increased sweating, blushing or somesuch.

The idea of motivated forgetting is the only theory of forgetting that mentions the person who is forgetting. The general argument is that certain memories become inaccessible to recall because of the way in which they relate to personal problems. The memories are not recalled because if they were they would be in some way unacceptable to the person; they might produce anxiety, guilt or some other unpleasant emotion in the person.

To some extent an understanding of motivated forgetting is helped by a knowledge of *amnesia*, which seems to be the limiting case of motivated forgetting. Typically, the amnesic forgets only items of personal reference such as his name or the whereabouts of his home. It has been found that amnesia is often preceded by a severe emotional shock suffered by the individual and from which the amnesia provides an escape. If you cannot remember who you are then you also cannot remember that you are the person who suffered and has to face such a terrible experience.

Although the idea of motivated forgetting makes good sense in everyday experience, it is impossible to speculate meaningfully about the degree to which it occurs consciously or unconsciously. Also it has proved extremely difficult to study in the laboratory. Reasons for this are obvious; it is very difficult to subject people to experiences which are sufficiently motivating to cause the necessary effects. However, there is one early and very influential exception to this. Zeigarnik (1927) gave subjects a series of complicated puzzles to solve and difficult tasks to do. Half of these tasks and problems she interrupted before they had been completed. Thereafter she simply tested her subjects' retention of the tasks. She found a very strong tendency to remember far more of the *uncompleted* than the completed tasks. These and similar experiments show that absorption in a task sets a strong motivation towards its completion and if this motive is unresolved through interruption it heightens memory for the task in question. If remembering can be motivated in this way, then there is little doubt that forgetting can be as well.

Decay Theory

Decay or disuse theory of memory depends very much on the idea of the *memory trace*, about which it is worth saying a little in the way of general background. It is very easy to assume that if traces of memory are spoken of then these actually exist; they have a physical entity. This may or may not be so. At present, the memory trace is an entirely hypothetical entity. Even though it is known that certain chemicals and chemical transmitters in the brain have something to do with learning and memory, it is still not possible to point to a memory trace in the brain. In hypothetical terms, it merely refers to whatever it is in the brain that represents an experience that can be recalled. If, as in decay theory, it is said that the memory trace fades, this is really saying no more than that what emerges on recall is different from whatever was originally registered. The memory trace is a hypothetical construct, although the suggestion is that it does exist and that one day it may be possible to identify it.

One form of decay theory suggests that a memory trace is formed whenever a person has an experience and that this fades away with time until it might eventually disappear altogether. This may be the result of normal metabolic processes in the brain. This is a theory which puts together time and physiology and certainly seems to be reasonable subjectively. Its main support comes from the way in which barely learned material fades rapidly from memory, although there is *no direct evidence* for it. Although some forgetting may occur in this way, it most certainly cannot account for some of the phenomena of memory. For example, a person does not forget how to swim or to ride a bicycle even though he may not have done so for many years. And the old are notorious for raising memories of very early experiences that they have not thought of for many years. Also people forget less if they sleep for several hours following learning than if they stay awake. Decay theory can account for none of these effects. For example, the theory *must* predict that 20 years without swimming would be ample time for the memory traces to decay through disuse; and it would be very unlikely that the person would have been engaging in any form of mental rehearsal of swimming during this time.

An alternative view of the decay theory is that, rather than fading with time, the memory trace becomes systematically distorted. Again, emphasis is placed on an interaction between time and physiological change whereby a memory loss is produced by spontaneous but orderly changes in the brain. It has been well established with pictorial material and stories, that memories do distort systematically. They tend to become more symmetrical, irregularities are accentuated and assimilations are made to other things which resemble the original source. But such distortions do not go with the mere passage of time. Some distortions occur when the figure is first reproduced or the story is first retold, and then later reproductions and retellings reflect the first distortions. So, again, for this variant of decay theory there is no direct supporting evidence.

The one way in which ideas of memory based on time and physiological change have some force is that which is concerned with *consolidation* theory. Here, the argument is that the memory trace needs some time to consolidate in the brain before it becomes firmly entrenched. If this process is interrupted in some way then forgetting is far more likely to occur. Much of the evidence for this idea comes from research into the effects of electro-convulsive shock (ECS). This is a mild electric shock which is passed across the heads of certain patients suffering from extreme depression and similar disorders. Although painless, its immediate effects are to produce a mild convulsion and then unconsciousness. Although it seems to help in some cases of depression, it produces complete forgetting of immediately preceding events.

Results similar to this have been found in studies with animals; there is less retention after ECS, particularly if it is given immediately after learning. Also, retention can be hindered by giving immediate injections of chemicals that interfere with protein synthesis. And finally, similar effects have sometimes been observed with what might be called emotional shock; for example, firing an unexpected pistol shot immediately after learning. All of which evidence is usually interpreted as suggesting that the memory trace needs some time to consolidate and that if this is hampered then retention is impaired. Although being relevant to an understanding of the physiological substrates of memory, work such as this neither proves nor disproves decay theory, which remains in a state of never having been directly tested in properly controlled conditions. Perhaps it is impossible to do so.

Interference (Inhibition) Theory

The basic idea of the interference theory of memory is that interference or inhibition from some learning leads to the forgetting of other learned material. Its status can best be summarised by stating that there is good evidence that it accounts for some forgetting, but apparently not for all.

Many of the studies which derive from this theory have been concerned with *retroactive interference*; this refers to the obvious case of *new* learning interfering with retention of *previously* learned material. The typical way in which this has been studied is according to a very straightforward experimental procedure involving two groups of subjects.

| Experimental group | Learn A | Learn B | Recall A |
| Control group | Learn A | Rest | Recall A |

(A and B might refer to two lists of words, to tennis and squash, or indeed to virtually anything.)

Both groups learn the first material, then whilst the experimental group learn the second material, the control group rests (does nothing) for the same period of time and finally both groups are tested on the original material. If the control group recall better than the experimental group then it can be inferred that the learning of B has interfered retroactively with the retention of A in the experimental group.

The obvious variable which has been most often manipulated in this procedure is the amount or nature of the interpolated activity or material for the experimental group. In this way, the amount of forgetting which occurs in a given time interval can be controlled. As might be expected, the general rule is that interpolated material which is most similar to the original leads to most interference and hence the greatest deleterious effects on retention.

There is one problem with this procedure; the control group always forgets something. Is this due to decay over time or to some type of interference? Retroactive interference theory can only account for this if ordinary waking life can be seen as corresponding in some respects to the active learning of material B which occurs between the original learning and eventual recall in the experimental group. One way of attempting to test this is by making the control group *sleep* during its rest period. Clearly, it is difficult to achieve precise control over when someone sleeps, but some studies have come near to it and have confirmed that more is remembered under these conditions, particularly with rote rather than organised materials.

As was mentioned above, it is very difficult to disprove a decay theory and therefore virtually impossible to carry out critical studies which would distinguish between this and retroactive interference. Some studies with cockroaches have come nearest, in which the cockroaches were put into a state of suspended animation immediately after learning. Under these conditions there was very little drop in retention, a result which supports retroactive interference theory but which does not disprove decay theory. Also, of course, memory in a cockroach may be a far cry from memory in a human.

As well as interference occuring retroactively, old memories may interfere with the retention of new material; this is termed *proactive interference.* The experimental procedure for testing this is very similar to that for retroactive interference, although differing in one important element.

Experimental group	Learn A	Learn B	Recall B
Control group	Rest	Learn B	Recall B

Whilst the experimental group is learning material A, the control group rests for the same period of time. Then both groups go on to learn B and to be tested on its retention.

Again, if the recall of the experimental group is worse than that of the control group, it can be inferred that the learning of A has interfered proactively (in a forward direction) with the recall of B which was learned later. The amount of proactive interference increases from the material in the two conditions being most similar to it being most dissimilar.

Of course, in real life these two types of interference doubtless have their effects simultaneously and it is quite clear that interference theory in general does account for a great deal of forgetting. It is the best supported theory with a great deal of evidence to back it up. On the other hand, it is impossible to entirely rule out the possibility of a passive decay of memory over time. Also, there is sufficient evidence that motivated forgetting occurs and can perhaps be used to explain some individual differences in forgetting, so as not to leave this out of consideration either. It may well be that in part each of these three ways of viewing forgetting has some substance to it and that an eventual theory must have elements in it from each of them.

Eidetic Imagery

A final word must be given to those individuals who appear to violate all the rules and generalisations about memory and forgetting mentioned so far in this chapter. These are the fortunate people who have what is commonly known as photographic memories and who are known by psychologists as having eidetic imagery. Such people can quite literally look briefly at a page of a book and then reproduce it exactly, as though they were scanning an internal photograph. Their problem would seem to be one of what and how to forget rather than what and how to remember, as is the case for most of us.

Although at present little can be said about eidetic imagers — they seem to be born rather than made, even though it is possible to train memory to be more efficient — it is perhaps worth describing the extremity to which their interesting abilities may sometimes go. Most people are familiar with stereoscopes in which the illusion of three dimensions (depth) is produced by presenting slightly different views of the same scene to the two eyes. There is a famous series of drawings sometimes used to study such effects in perception each of which is made up of an amazingly complex series of thousands of dots. When the two views of these are put together stereoscopically then certain figures and designs are seen, which cannot otherwise be picked out of the patterns.

If one view of such a figure is presented on a particular day to the left eye of an eidetic imager and then some days or even weeks later the other view is presented to the right eye, he can 'read off' the figure which can only be seen stereoscopically. The precision and amount of detail recalled to allow this is incredible. Doubtless, research into the rare eidetic imagers in the world will eventually further knowledge of memory even if it can tell us little of forgetting.

Summary Points

(1) There are various types of remembering, these being in order of ease: relearning, recognition, and recall.
(2) The early work on memory was concerned with the study of 'pure' memory, making much use of the nonsense syllable, and paired-associate and serial learning. Concern has also centred on systematic distortions which can occur in memory and on the study of mnemonics which show memory to be a matter of active organisation.
(3) More recent work on memory has dwelt on four main systems or processes. (a) Sensory information storage which is concerned with the first few milliseconds of experience in which sensory information is stored in iconic form. (b) Short term memory which lasts for approximately 18 seconds. (c) Long term memory into which items pass from short term memory as they are rehearsed and on which much research has focused, although a great deal remains to be done. (d) Retrieval: the process by which items stored in memory are made available.
(4) Forgetting tends to follow a smooth course in most cases. There are three main theories to explain it. (a) That which suggests that forgetting is motivated and concentrates on individual differences. (b) That which links time and physiological change and suggests that memories simply decay with time. (c) That which sees forgetting as a matter of the interference of some learning with the retention of other material. Each of these theories has something to be said for it and may be necessary to an eventual more inclusive theory. At present there is more support for the interference theory than for the others, although it clearly cannot account for all aspects of forgetting.
(5) Eidetic imagers are those people with apparently photographic memories; they transgress all the established rules of memory.

Study Questions – 5

(1) Patients in hospital are (usually) in a very unfamiliar setting. Do you think that they become disoriented by this so that their memory is im-

paired? What other aspects of being ill might affect memory?

(2) In what ways might a change in a person's physical state of condition, be it temporary or permanent, affect his memory? Do you think that your own memory is affected by such things as fatigue or alcohol?

(3) In the caring professions it is often necessary to remember important items or even to get patients to do the same. If you have not done so already, work out some mnemonic devices to aid in this.

(4) Try to find some examples from your professional training and duties of retroactive and proactive interference.

(5) During the course of caring for your patients it is almost inevitable that you have forgotten some parts of your training. Why have you forgotten these parts and not others?

(6) Find everyday hospital examples of forgetting and extinction. What are the similarities and differences between the two processes?

(7) In 'explaining' why he has forgotten something, a person will often say, 'It's just my bad memory'. Do you think that it is reasonable for him to speak of his memory in this way, as though it were a separate entity, out of his control?

(8) How would you train yourself to improve your memory for your own study materials and in your professional life? Would your scheme work for other people?

(9) In what ways could you make use of the fact that it is easier to relearn something than to recognise it and easier to recognise it than to recall it?

(10) To what extent do you think that memory and forgetting are motivated? List examples from your training of things you have found it easy to remember and those you have forgotten too easily. Do you think that your own interests have motivated this?

6 PERCEPTION

The psychology of perception is concerned with the detailed and precise analysis of a set of processes which are integral to behaviour. All organisms are constantly bombarded with stimuli, both from without and from within. There would be no advantage in attending to and processing all these stimuli and in any case it is unlikely that any organism has the capacity so to do. Perception then amounts to the selection of some stimuli and the ignoring of others, and then the transformation of those selected into meaningful and useful information.

The processing of information allows the organism to make predictions about the world and thereby helps to minimise surprise, which in turn presents a more harmonious interaction with the world than would otherwise be possible. Although it would seem that a necessary fore-runner of information processing is that an organism has the ability to sense the incoming stimuli, it has proved of little use to psychologists to distinguish between the characteristics of sensation and those of perception; they are simply parts of the same overall process. No attempt will be made to distinguish between them here.

As will become obvious below, perceptual research often progresses by the construction of theoretical models which can be tested to see how well they represent reality. These models usually take the implicit form of – 'it seems *as if* perceptual process X is like . . . if so, then what follows?' In their 'as if' qualities, theoretical models should be distinguished from theories which posit that the world is 'as' something or the other. It remains to see how well such models of perceptual processes do reflect reality.

(Note: In this chapter I shall be discussing only visual perception. Perceptual mechanisms are linked to each of the five senses, but it is usual to exemplify research into perception, with vision, since this is the most complex system and psychologists have spent correspondingly longer in analysing it.)

Recognition of Patterns

As an example of one of the most basic and important perceptual processes, that of dealing with sensory information, the fundamental matter of how patterns are recognised will be discussed. Pattern recognition is a capacity which is so integral to perceptual ability that it is easy to take it for granted, but a little thought will show what a complex matter it must be.

Template matching. The simplest model of pattern recognition is that of so-called template matching, which implies that we recognise patterns by matching a perceptual image of something against an internal representation (a template) of it. If it matches then we accept and name it, if not, we reject it and match it with another representation. Although at first sight this seems a reasonable way of conceptualising pattern recognition, it is in fact clumsy. It means that we must have a template not only for each set of stimuli, but also for each stimulus in any orientation or for any slight change in shape, colour, size, etc. in which it might be presented to us. Such a scheme has the unwieldy qualities of the Chinese alphabet. One cannot infer from this argument that patterns are not matched in this way, merely that it is very unlikely that they are.

Preprocessing. An alternative view is that which suggests that a stimulus pattern is preprocessed into some standard form which is then matched against the appropriate templates. This is again possible, but it is still a clumsy scheme which can lead to many potential perceptual errors and which leaves questions unanswered. For example, it cannot deal with how new patterns are processed, and it says little of how the preprocessing might occur.

Illusions. An important way in which attempts have been made to understand pattern recognition is through a consideration of the perceptual errors that are made when people are beguiled by illusions. These are exemplified in Figure 6.1. From such illusions it may be seen that pattern perception is influenced both by *critical features* of the stimuli (line, intersection, angle size, etc.) or the *context* in which they occur.

Also relevant here are reversible figures (see Figure 6.2), of which it is possible to make two interpretations, but only one at a time, even though the two might follow close on each other, the figure seeming to slip back and forth. Study the staircase or cornice in the illustration for example. If you are honest with yourself, you will realise that it is impossible to make both interpretations of it simultaneously. Such figures suggest that any pattern can be interpreted in many ways. So it is argued that on being presented with a pattern we form an hypothesis about it based on some of its salient features; we then test this and accept or reject it according to the test. If we reject it, then we form

Figure 6.1 Visual Illusions

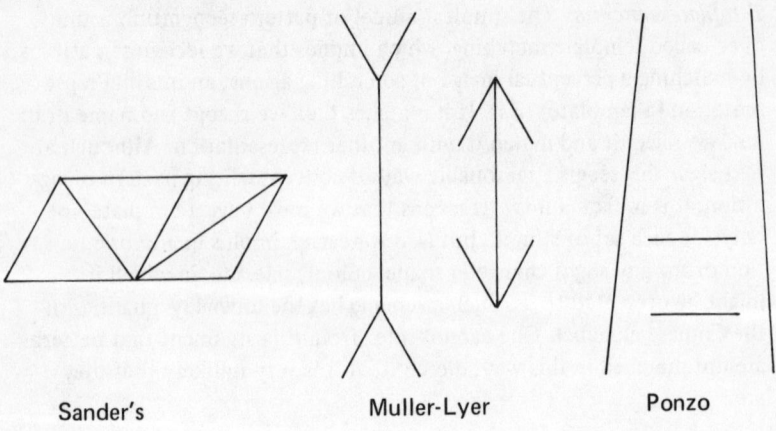

Sander's   Muller-Lyer   Ponzo

Figure 6.2 Reversible Figure: Staircase/Cornice

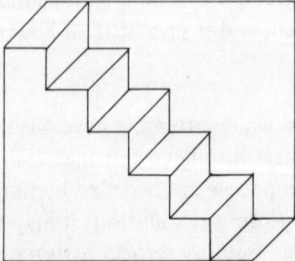

another hypothesis. This idea highlights the inaccuracy of many of our perceptions.

In this context, a final clue to understanding is given by impossible figures (see Figure 6.3). These suggest that basic pattern recognition must be integrated, that is, to be meaningful objects must be perceived within a known context.

Information Processing

The ideas discussed above have led to the development of a number of principles of human information processing; principles which are thought to be at the heart of pattern recognition.

Figure 6.3 Impossible Trident

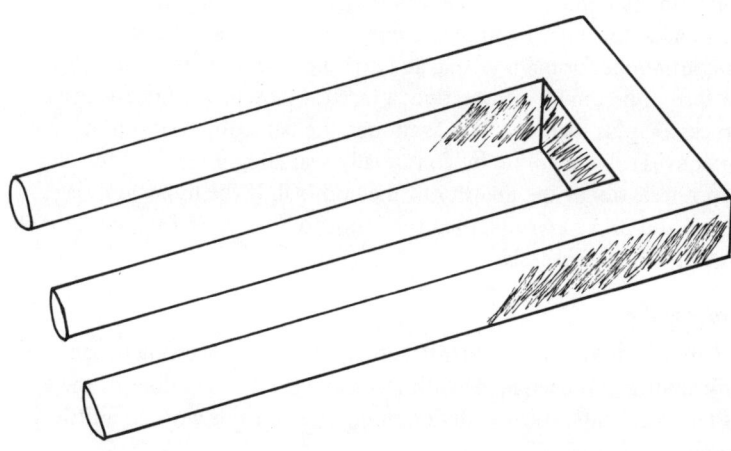

(1) Perception is interpretative;

(2) perception is active;

(3) perception occurs over time, it is not just instantaneous;

(4) perception involves an extraction of the critical features of the stimuli under regard;

(5) perception involves the organisation of these figures into consistent meaningful patterns;

(6) perception is accurate only if interpretation fits any contextual information into consistent images.

Analysis by Synthesis

One of the most promising discussions of pattern recognition to follow on from the above can be found in Neisser (1967) and Lindsay and Norman (1972); it is known as analysis by synthesis. The thesis begins with the suggestion that we analyse the features of the energy patterns which impinge on our sense organs. The results of this analysis are then thought to pass into a memory store in which they are also interpreted. All of which occurs in a few parts of a second. In this system the answer to the problem of how we recognise patterns is thought to come from a knowledge of stimuli which have been interpreted and recognised, this leading in turn to expectations concerning the next message from the sense organs.

As these expectations change, it is argued that an active synthesising begins, a process which is speeded up or slowed down by the context in which the stimuli occur. The process is faster if the relevant stimuli are appearing in a familiar and hence predictable environment. To summarise this rather complex theory, analysis by synthesis is a process of continuous forming, testing and revising of hypotheses about the pattern of incoming information; a mixture of sensory and cognitive processes, plus memory. It is as though the perceptual capacities were detectives solving crimes by continually searching their clues to form hypotheses about the identity of the criminal. If the hypothesis is tested and proved wrong, then they turn to their clues for another look and another hypothesis.

Frogs and Cats

A very instructive and influential analysis of the processing of sensory information has been made with research into the functions of the eyes of frogs and cats. It is worth describing some of this work in a little detail.

Lettvin et al.(1959) embedded electrodes into various parts of the optic nerves of frogs and then exposed the animals to many patterns of visual stimuli. From the responses they measured they were able to conclude that the frog can extract four different patterns of information from visual stimuli, each corresponding to its own type of detector in the eye. It can detect: (a) edges; light/dark borders, (b) movement and contrast; moving edges or borders, (c) dimming, a lowering in overall illumination, and (d) convex edges; small dark, circular, moving objects, i.e. 'bug' detection.

These complex detections are made in the retina of the eye, although even this degree of retinal complexity would not be good enough for the complex perceptions of man. In fact, even the frog will die when surrounded by flies, *if the flies do not move*. Its neural template sets it only for moving flies. Overall, it can be concluded from this work on the frog's eye that the frog's brain does not receive basic, crude information, or even a one-to-one translation of whatever patterns of light strike the retina. Some processing goes on before any information is passed to the Central Nervous System.

Moving on to the cat's eye, this has a simple retinal organisation but one which occurs in stages. Summarising an important and difficult series of experiments carried out by Hubel and Wiesel (e.g. 1965), the cat processes visual information by apparently answering a series of questions such as the following: (a) Is there a contour present? (b) Is this contour an edge or a line? (c) If it is a line, is it against a light or a dark background? (d) What is its orientation? (e) Is it moving? (f) If it is moving, then in what direction? (g) What angle does it subtend? (h) What then is its size?

At the human level, the neural networks which allow the processing of visual features are very complex and sophisticated. Although it is known that, as in the frog and cat, visual feature detectors exist in man, what exactly they are and how they work is unclear. However, the type of findings described above promise well for possible application at the human level.

Complex Perceptual Functions of Man

Discussion so far has centred on the processing of sensory information. In man, this processing takes a number of varied and complex forms, some of the more important of which will be described below.

Brightness

An awareness of changes in brightness is perhaps the simplest visual experience. It depends on three factors, (a) the intensity of light striking a particular part of the retina, (b) the intensity of light recently experienced – adaptation, and (c) the intensity of light striking surrounding areas of the retina – contrast.

The two important processes involved here are adaptation and contrast. Imagine your visual experiences on going into a darkened cinema; you slowly become used to the dark and gradually begin to see more of your surroundings. In fact, the adaptation is not quite as gradual as it seems to be. It takes the form shown in Figure 6.4.

The reason for the double curve is that two processes are involved in dark adaptation. The cone cells of the retina adapt first, taking about seven minutes, and then the rod cells continue to adapt for more than an hour. The only exception to this is if you enter a room illuminated with dim red light. In this environment, the rods do not adapt at all.

An example of the effect of simultaneous brightness *contrast* is given in Figure 6.5. The small grey square on the left *looks* brighter than that on the right even though they are of the same brightness. This effect occurs through a process of interaction in the visual neurons; it is termed lateral inhibition. This simply means that the activity of one visual cell is modified by the activity of cells adjacent to it, a process which allows us to have greater acuity for detail and the perception of contours.

Figure 6.4 Dark Adaptation Curve

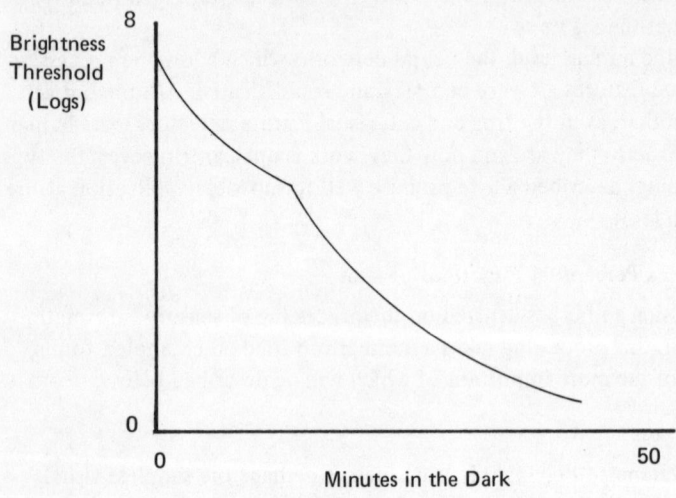

Figure 6.5 Simultaneous Brightness Contrast

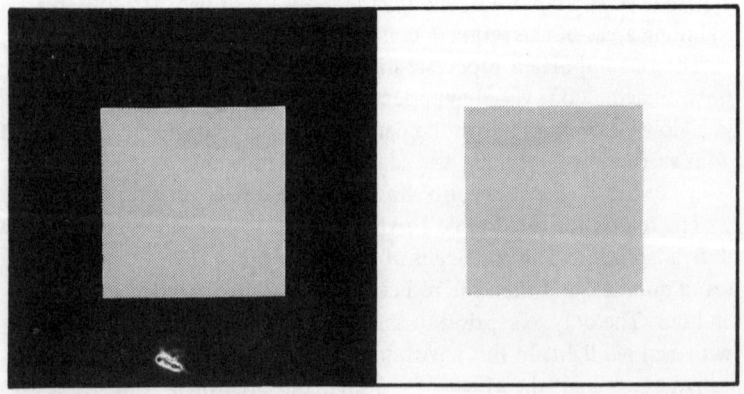

Acuity

There are various measures of visual acuity (perceptual sharpness or keenness). It is a process which involves detecting, naming, discriminating and localising an object. Acuity is one of the main visual capacities tested by the optician. For example, if you have 20/20 vision this means that at 20 feet you can see what a normal eye can, whereas if you have 20/200 vision you can only see at 20 feet what a normal eye can see at 200 feet.

There can be various disorders of acuity, the most common of which is *myopia.* This is commonly known as near-sightedness, distant objects appearing blurred. Its cause is an elongation of the eyeball which leads images to be focused in front of the surface of the retina rather than on it (where they should be for perfect acuity). *Hyperopia*, on the other hand, is far-sightedness, involving a blurring of near objects and caused by a flattening of the eyeball which leads to images being focused behind the retinal surface.

Finally, *temporal acuity* should be mentioned. If you see a brief flash of light, the image of this persists for 150-250 milliseconds. So, at a certain rate (15-16 flashes per second) which is termed the critical fusion frequency, a flashing light will appear to be continuous. This is temporal acuity.

Perception of Depth

The main question which psychologists have asked about the perception of depth is — how can the brain take a flat image from each eye and put these together so that depth is experienced? The answer is that the brain is aided in this by two types of cues, binocular (two eyed) and monocular (one eyed).

To deal first with the binocular cues, these begin with *binocular parallax.* As the eyes are at different points in the head they provide slightly different pictures of the world, as is the case with a stereoscope. The fusion of these two pictures in the brain (for which there must be specialised detectors) is sufficient for the perception of depth. Related to this is *motion parallax.* There are differences in the displacement of the representation of a moving object across the retina with distance, and this of course will be slightly different for each eye, again aiding the perception of depth. Also, the eyes *converge* (rotate inwards) more when viewing a near object than one far away. The muscular feedback from this gives another cue to depth.

Binocular and monocular cues to depth come together with the phenomenon of *accommodation.* As the distance of an object changes so the lens of the eye(s) changes thickness in order to maintain focus. Again, feedback from the muscles which create this change gives a cue to distance/depth.

Monocular cues to depth or distances are more straightforward than binocular cues and can be listed easily. (a) *Size* — the further away an object is, the smaller it appears. (b) *Overlap* — nearby objects often partly obscure objects which are farther away. (c) *Shadows* — their size and length make an obvious contribution to depth perception. (d) *Pers-*

pective — in linear perspective parallel lines converge with distance and the amount of detail which can be perceived decreases with distance in an orderly gradient of texture; in aerial perspective, with distance all objects become greyer. Each of these monocular cues to depth can only work in one way. For example, a far object can never partly obscure a near object, and, of course, these cues can have their effects with only one eye being used.

Colour

The way in which colour is perceived is an extraordinarily complex matter and will therefore be touched upon but briefly. In broad terms, three dimensions are necessary to represent colour: brightness (intensity), hue (dominance of light wavelength), and saturation (purity in white light). In the light spectrum only three colours are primary (pure), red, green, and blue. A mixing of these in various combinations and proportions leads to all the other colours in an additive way, clearly a very different process than that involved in mixing coloured paints, this being subtractive. Some people are colour-blind, this more commonly being restricted to red/green or blue/yellow blindness. It is very rare to find a person who is totally colour blind, that is one who can only, like dogs, perceive black and white.

These, and many similar facts have led to a number of intricate theories of colour vision. One such theory states that we have three types of receptor for colour, namely for red, green or blue respectively. And another, the opponent-process theory, suggests that there are three types of coding mechanism, for red-green, blue-yellow and black-white respectively. The most intricate theory combines the two already mentioned to posit that there are three types of receptor in the cone cells of the retina, the information from which is combined in the brain by inhibitory opponent processes. Here is not the place to describe these theories in greater detail.

Organisation in Perception

The nature of organisational processes in perception revives the earlier discussion of analysis by synthesis, or the continuous forming and testing of hypothesis about incoming information. If it is reasonable to construe perceptual experiences as proceeding in this way, then it becomes meaningless to attempt to draw distinctions between sensations and perception. Indeed, to carry the argument a stage further it becomes artificial and overly contrived to make distinctions between perception and cognition and memory, since the latter are also concerned with the processing of information, although more particularly with its meaning.

The usual way of construing these complicated mental processes is that they involve a continual transformation of information into various codes. Only some of this information is extracted and organised. There are a number of hypothetical models of how these processes might occur, notably those described by Neisser (1967) and Sperling (1967). Discussion of some of these can be found in Chapter 5 on memory and cognition.

Whilst recognising that to some extent a distinction between perceptual and cognitive organisation is arbitrary, some organisation matters have traditionally been placed in the perceptual domain. A description of the more important ideas on perceptual organisation will follow.

Figural Organisation

A prerequisite to the perception of form and shape is that the characteristics of the contours of a figure are coded directly into individual cells within the visual system of the brain. Two aspects of figural organisation deserve particular mention: the ability to perceive a figure as distinct from its background, and the Gestalt laws of perceptual organisation.

A figure contains contours which define its particular form and shape. How do we perceive this form? How can we pick out the figure from its background? Early work on the so-called *ganzfeld* gave the lead to an answer to these questions. If you were to place half a table-tennis ball over each eye the result would be that you would appear to be looking out into a completely homogeneous field; there is no way of distinguishing one part of it from another. Some subjects say that it is like looking out into a dense fog, and others say that their visual experiences have stopped altogether. Thus, for perception of form to occur at all there must be changes in both space and time.

This work on the ganzfeld was extended by research involving *stabilised retinal images*. When we look at some object fixedly, our eyes in fact are not perfectly still. They move back and forth rapidly, a phenomenon known as physiological nystagmus. Equipment has been devised which stops this movement, thus allowing the image which strikes the retina to remain precisely in one place. Under these conditions subjects report that the image of the object they are fixating gradually fades away. In order to maintain organisation in perception, we need *change* in retinal stimulation. Sometimes this change comes about through movement in the world and always it is created by the continual to and fro movements of our eyes.

It was in the 1920s to 1940s that a group of mainly German psychologists put forward certain laws of perceptual organisation, and even though several decades have passed their status as laws is undiminished. These *Gestalt* laws are as follows:

(a) Pregnanz. Perceptions are organised so that they seem simple and orderly. Perception organises in the direction of simplicity, symmetry and ease of memory.

(b) Proximity. The elements of an array of stimuli tend to be grouped perceptually. For example, we always see xx xx xx as three double xxs and not as six single xs or two triple xs.

(c) Similarity. Similar elements in an array of stimuli are perceived as a group. For example, when looking at a muddled set of objects we would tend to group all the square objects together perceptually and distinguish them from all the circular objects.

(d) Continuity/common fate. Elements in a set of stimuli tend to be grouped together if they are oriented in a particular direction or if they are moving in a common direction.

(e) Closure. Parts of any figures which are missing tend to be filled in perceptually so that they form a whole. Thus we perceive ⟨⟩ as a full circle and not as a series of unrelated dashes.

Each of these descriptions of organisation processes is the outcome of perceptual interpretation.

Spatial Organisation

The matter of how we organise our perception of space has already been partly discussed. Cues to depth perception are all part of the perceptual organisation of space. Understanding of spatial organisation has been ingeniously extended by Ames (e.g. 1951). His experimental procedure involved the construction of highly distorted rooms with strangely sloping and oddly sized floors and walls, the precise construction being carried out in such a way that on looking into the room the observer has cues to depth which are systematically different from that which they would be normally. Thus of two people standing in the room, the nearer one actually looks further away to the observer than the more distant one.

From a series of such demonstrations, which are very dramatic, Ames argues that our perceptions of the world are in reality *assumptions* which are based on whatever information is available at the time, *plus* past experience. On viewing Ames' room, subjects *assume* that, like other rooms, it is rectangular, and since in reality it is not, they see the persons within as of the wrong sizes and hence as standing at different distances. Psychologists who support this assumptive view of perceptual organisation are known as transactionalists, arguing that perception is the result of a transaction between a person and his environment.

Constancies

Past experience also enters very much into what are known as the perceptual constancies. When we see objects, we do not perceive them as they actually are, nor do we in some way observe the images they cast on our retinas. We perceive them with the *aid* of retinal images. The information this image passes on is processed and internal representations of the world are constructed. For the most part these perceptions are fairly accurate and do not change much over time; they remain stable. This stability is known as constancy.

There are various types of constancy, of brightness, colour, shape, size, and so on. If we see someone whom we know well and know to be of six feet in height and he is 50 yards away, then we still see him as six feet in height, not as much smaller. If we were judging his height simply through a processing of the image of him as it struck our retinas, then we would perceive him as very small.

To take another example, we perceive the tops of tables as being square or rectangular — we *know* them to be this shape. But it is very rarely that we look down on a table top from directly above; normally we see it at such an angle that the shape which is actually represented in the retinal image is that of a distorted trapezoid. And for one final example, if you own a car or live in a house, and you see either of these at night you will perceive them in their usual colours. In fact, there will be very little colour present in the retinal image; constancy is organising your perceptions.

That the perceptual constancies depend very much upon past experience is demonstrated by a consideration of the perception of unfamiliar objects. It is very difficult to judge their size, shape, colour, brightness or distance. Consider again the example of making observations at night and reflect how difficult it is to perceive the colour of an unfamiliar cat. All cats look grey at night — unless you know them. So, we do not take the image on our retinas and translate it directly; we perceive some compromise between this and our knowledge of the object in question. Whether this capacity is built-in to us or we have to learn it is still unresolved within psychology. One final point which it is worth making about perceptual constancy is that it is a capacity which has to be suspended by successful artists. To represent the world they have to push out constancies and rely solely upon their retinal images. They express this in two dimensions and on viewing the result our constancies allow us to perceive in three dimensions, familiar shapes, and so on.

Selectivity

Perceptual

As was mentioned previously, perceptions are selective; they have to be. Imagine attempting to exist if you perceived every stimulus in your immediate environment equally. Nothing would stand out, all would be equal and there would be no meaning attached to anything. Perception must be, and is, selective, but such selectivity brings with it an enormous problem. If selectivity is to work, then *all* stimuli must first be recognised and then some of them discarded; it seems that some type of censor mechanism has to be at work.

This hypothetical censoring mechanism has been conceptualised in two major ways. The first is known as *active filtering* (Broadbent, 1958), in which it is argued that some information is blocked at one level of perception so that whatever is blocked does not reach the next level. This idea places the selectivity process in the perceptual mechanism. The alternative view, *active processing*, places the selectivity at the more cognitive level with the suggestion that some aspects of the world are simply ignored and hence drop out of awareness.

Work on the ways in which perception is selective has gone ahead in a number of spheres. One of the more interesting of these, known as *visual search*, owes much to Neisser (e.g. 1964), for its development. In visual search experiments, subjects are simply given long lists of letters to scan through in search of particular target items. Much basic information has been gathered using this technique. For example, looking for the presence of a letter is faster than looking for its absence; more processing occurs when a critical item is embedded in every line of the list. Looking for a 'Q' in a background of circular letters is harder than seeking it in a context of angular letters; which means that more processing is needed when a target item has features similar to those of the items in its context. And finally, after practice, searching for ten items is just as fast and easy as searching for one item.

Subjects make these visual searches at high speeds, thereby showing that we can select information that we require without analysing every bit of it that is available.

Understanding of selectivity in perception has also increased through research into the way in which subjects *look at pictures*, particularly if these are unfamiliar. This research relies on a complex photographic technique which allows a recording to be made of a subject's eye-fixations as he looks at a picture.

When looking at pictures, our eyes do not follow a smooth and orderly series of movements. They jump rapidly from point to point, on each of which they dwell for a few moments. The film recordings of such eye movements show that unpredictable and unusual contours are fixated much more than are the familar and predictable. It is as though there is an active search being made for variation. Information which is coming in from peripheral vision (that which the subject glimpses from the corner of his eyes) is apparently guiding the choice of what next he fixates. Also, and of course more complicatedly, this peripheral information is determining where *not* to look next.

In a sense, ideas which have stemmed from visual search and eye fixations on looking at unfamiliar pictures come together with research into the perceptual or cognitive aspects of reading. To use the terms of academic psychology, reading involves a search for multiple targets and the recognition of letters and words. Film recordings have shown that when reading, the eyes fixate every 250/300 milliseconds and make small saccadic movements every 25/50 milliseconds. Also, reading is not the smooth left-to-right progression of the eyes that it might appear to be; there are large numbers of regressive movements. All of which indicates that the movements of the eyes during reading are dependent on information gained from their previous fixation – somehow they are commanded by information which is not yet fully in awareness.

Cognitive

Although, as already mentioned, a precise distinction between perception and cognition is impossible, and probably undesirable, it is reasonable to point to broad differences between perception and related higher mental processes such as thinking and motivation. Although full discussion of this is made elsewhere, it is important now to mention ways in which cognitive processes contribute to the selective nature of perception. In brief, our perceptions can be influenced by motivation (including our bodily needs) by values and by personal and social factors. These influences will be exemplified in turn.

Most people will have had the experience of being very hungry and catching sight of many objects in the environment which seem either to be food or to be related to food, only to be disappointed when examining them more closely. This type of sensitisation has been confirmed in the laboratory with that widely used perceptual apparatus – the tachistoscope. This is a device which enables visual stimuli to be presented to subjects for very brief but exactly controlled durations. Subjects deprived of food for some hours perceive food related words much faster (that is, at briefer exposure times) than they perceive non-food-related words of similar familiarity and frequency in the language (e.g. Wispe and Dramarean, 1953).

In 1947, Bruner and Goodman carried out a fascinating and much quoted study on the influence of needs on perception. Although very dramatic and convincing it should be borne in mind that it has not been successfully repeated, so its status is a little in doubt. Bruner and Goodman studied ten to eleven year old children, some of whom came from prosperous homes, others from slums. They set them the task of adjusting the size of a variable circular opening until they judged it to be equal to the size of certain coins. Sometimes they did this from memory and sometimes with the coin in front of them.

The results showed that the children overestimated the sizes of the coins, the amount of overestimation increasing with the value of the coins, and the poorer children overestimated more than the richer. In Bruner and Goodman's view, this proved a definite relationship between needs, values and perceptual selectivity.

That values in themselves can influence perception was demonstrated by Postman, Bruner and McGinnies (1948). They gave their subjects a questionnaire designed to measure the extent to which they valued things religious, social, economic, aesthetic, political, and theoretical. They then used a tachistoscope to show the subjects a series of words, some to do with these six areas of concern, others not. In general, subjects had faster recognition times for words which were concerned with those areas which they particularly valued.

Possibly the most interesting motivational influence on perception comes with *perceptual defence* (see Eriksen and Eriksen, 1972, for a good analysis), in which the problem concerns stimuli which subjects seem highly motivated *not* to perceive. The study of perceptual defence which made the first impact was that of McGinnies (1949). He simply showed subjects a mixture of words one at a time tachistoscopically.

Some of these words were emotionally loaded, often obscene, and others were emotionally neutral.

The results of McGinnies' study seemed to bear out three important points. First, the emotionally disturbing stimuli had higher recognition thresholds than the neutral words, that is subjects needed to see them for much longer exposure times before they recognised them. Second, the emotional words so altered perceptions that often they were not recognised at all. And third, even though they were not recognised, these words aroused emotional reactions. This third point is at the nub of the problem of perceptual defence: how can a stimulus not be recognised and yet be recognised (in some sense it must have been recognised for the emotional response to be provoked)? Stated more generally, how can a person avoid perceiving a stimulus *before* he has actually perceived what it is?

At first it was thought that results such as McGinnies' might have been spurious. For example, it might have been that the emotionally loaded words were of much lower frequency in the language than the neutral words; frequency is known to be related to recognition thresholds, the more frequent words being the more easily recognised. Alternatively, it might have been that subjects were simply embarrassed at reporting the obscene words to the experimenter and made doubly sure of what they were seeing before so reporting. However, subsequent studies showed similar perceptual defence effects with nonsense syllables that had previously been associated with electric shock, in comparison with those that had not.

The problem of perceptual defence remains unanswered. Recent studies have added greatly to the theoretical and empirical complexities of the matter, but whatever these complexities they must revolve around the basic problem of how a subject cannot perceive something without first perceiving it.

Finally, perception is affected, that is made more selective, by personal and social influences. As yet there is no all-embracing theory as to how these influences come about, so for the present they will just be illustrated. Witkin et al (1954) gave subjects a series of perceptual tasks designed to relate their personalities to perceptual responding. Many of these tasks involved placing subjects in chairs in rooms either of which could be tilted independently. The subject's task was to judge whether or not a line in front of him was vertical. Witkin found that his subjects could be distinguished as to whether they were field-dependent or field-independent. Field-dependent subjects made their judgements by using whatever information they could from their environment. Field-independent subjects judged on the basis of internal cues, presumably from their organs of balance. These subjects then seemed set to perceive the world in different ways by their basic personalities.

That social factors can influence perception was convincingly shown in a study by Asch (1951) which again required subjects to judge a line. A subject was brought to the laboratory with others whom he believed to be subjects like himself. His task was to call out a series of decisions about which of three comparison lines was equal in length to a standard line. He had to make his decision after the other subjects, who were in fact stooges of the experimenter.

After a few correct decisions, the stooges began systematically to distort their judgements and choose incorrect lines. Under these conditions a significant proportion of genuine subjects also changed their judgements. Questioned afterwards, some of these admitted changing their judgements because they did not wish to appear different from everyone else, even though they knew them to be wrong. More interestingly, others showed no awareness that they had been making incorrect judgements; their perceptions had been distorted without their knowledge by the pressure of social influence.

Summary Points

(1) Perception is concerned with the selection of stimuli from the vast numbers available, and with the translation of those selected into meaningful information.

(2) Pattern recognition exemplifies basic perceptual processes. Work on this and the perception of illusions and other unusual stimuli has led to the development of models of human information processing. One of the best of these applied to pattern recognition is analysis by synthesis, a viewpoint which sees perception as a constant testing of hypotheses.

(3) Various complex perceptual functions have been studied individually. These include perception of brightness, visual acuity, perception of depth, and the perception of colour.

(4) The matter of how perceptions are organised can be broken down into (a) figural organisation, which as work on the ganzfeld and the stabilised retinal image shows, depends on movement, and also on Gestalt principles; (b) spatial organisation, which is determined by perception of depth, possibly by assumptions that we make about the world, and (c) constancies, which refer to our perception being a compromise between retinal images and what we know of the object in question.

(5) The final set of problems in perception concerns selectivity. Our perceptions are not 'pure' but are influenced by some sort of filtering or processing as is shown by research into visual search, the viewing of pictures, and reading, and also by broader influences such as motivation and personal and social factors.

Study Questions – 6

(1) How would you test the perceptual capacities of a patient who could neither speak nor write?

(2) How might your perceptions of a hospital ward differ from those of a patient? How might a hungry person's perceptions differ from those of a person who had recently eaten?

(3) List any examples you can think of from your profession of people perceiving only what they want to perceive. How influential on perception is this factor?

(4) How might a person's bodily injuries influence his perceptions? How might they influence the way in which other people perceive him?

(5) How would you test whether or not a patient could perceive colour? Why might it be important to find this out?

(6) Can you imagine any professional situations in which you would need to alter or influence a patient's perceptions? How would you set about it?

(7) In the course of your work have you seen any everyday examples of perceptual defence? How do you think the process of perceptual defence comes about?

(8) In your concern to help a patient, what would be of more assistance to you: information about his perceptions or about his behaviour? Justify your answer.

(9) How can a one-eyed man perceive a three-dimensional world?

(10) List the ways in which your training has altered your perceptions. How might your perceptions differ from those of members of the other paramedical professions?

7 THINKING

Elements of Thinking

Like so many concepts in psychology, knowledge about thinking is gained by inference. It is impossible to be certain whether or not another person *is* thinking, irrespective of *what* he is thinking. This is obvious at the everyday level as well as in the psychological laboratory. We are used to guessing what other people are thinking, but it is never more than a guess. Consequently, in studying thinking the psychologist cannot be as objective as he would like to be. He has to ask questions and also to decide how much credence he gives to the answers he hears.

Also, to some extent, most thinking involves problem solving, unless of course it is sheer reverie or day-dreaming. Take an example of a relatively common stream of thoughts. Shortly after he starts a new job, a person is invited to dinner by his boss. This worries him and he gives it much thought. Why? He is unsure what his boss's motives are (generosity? a test? second thoughts about him?); he is unsure what clothes to wear (formal? casual?); he is unsure what sort of occasion it will be (formal/informal?, many other guests/none?); he is unsure about whether to be himself or to put on a facade.

All these thoughts have helped to *define* the problem. Next, his thoughts will take him in the direction of dredging up any *related* concepts he might have which will help in solving the problem. Hopefully, there will be long chains of verbally labelled concepts from previous learning. So he will go through any similar occasions he has experienced in the past and see what can be gained from them. Without such concepts he cannot properly define the problem. Naturally, this will not be the case in the above example, since he will have had some social experiences in his life. But this is by no means always the case. For example, I could not define a problem within the academic tradition of astronomy. I know nothing of its concepts.

Next, the man faced with the dinner party has to make decisions about the *relevance* of the concepts which have occurred to him. He must keep some concepts and discard others. He goes through all the social circumstances he has thought of and dwells more on those which seem relevant. For example, he might keep all those which have to do with evening meals, and all those in which he has met people whom he does not know well.

Finally, he has to construct *hypotheses* about which ideas are the key ones, and then go and *test* them. He might decide that, in the absence of any further information, he should regard his boss's motives as kindly rather than devious, that he had better dress fairly formally, that he should be properly courteous but otherwise behave normally, and that it would make very little difference how many people would be there. His thoughts will be put to the test when the time comes. This example has been dealt with in some detail since it represents the probable course of much of our thinking, although it may not seem as ordered as this to the man who is experiencing it.

Thinking then may be defined as: the manipulation of images and ideas, each of which are mental representations from experience.

To bridge the gap between mind and matter, it is clear that *muscle activity* is involved in thinking. Hess (1965), for example, has shown that when arithmetic problems are being solved, pupil size gradually increases, until solution, when there is contraction. The same is true of spelling. Also, if you ask someone to imagine an object, you will find his eye movements to be very similar to those he would make if he were actually examining the object. Similarly, the imagining of lifting a weight is correlated with patterns of action currents in the arm. And finally, heart rate often increases during problem solving, particularly when it is being done efficiently and particularly at critical moments. However, these apparent muscle components seem only to be a reflection of thinking, they are *not necessary* to it. If a person is given curare or any of its derivatives, his musculature is totally paralysed, but his thought processes are completely normal.

A related question concerns the extent to which *words* are necessary for thinking. Is thinking merely subvocal talking? Subjectively, this would often appear to be so and there was a great deal of early evidence that there is frequent electrical activity from the speech muscles whilst a person is thinking. Similarly, when a deaf person is thinking, there is a great deal of activity in his hands. However, such movements can only be regarded as concomitants of thought, although perhaps aiding it. They are not necessary to thinking, since there is clear evidence that animals and infants, neither of whom have language as we know it, can solve problems and hence (presumably) think.

Verbal Processes in Thinking

The above discussion leads onto a consideration of the general relationship between language and thought. If thinking is viewed as the manipulation of symbols which are sorted somewhere in the brain then it must involve processes such as recall, imagination, reasoning, understanding, etc. And language skills would be important in the manipulation of memory traces, if in no other way. Certainly, many studies have shown that 'talking to oneself' can help in problem-solving, seemingly verbal responses often *mediate* between concepts and action.

This type of mediation is essentially unobservable but it is obvious that words can be used to define a problem and to outline a possible response to it, before this response is ever made. 'I am uneasy. Why? I need to return home within the hour, it is raining and I have no coat. What to do? I'll wait until the last possible moment and if it has stopped raining all well and good; if not I can beg a lift from X.' The problem, simple though it is, has been defined and solved with words and no actions.

It is often the case that if a person faced with a problem is asked to say aloud what his plan of campaign will be then he will do better at the problem than will someone who has been allowed to keep his plan to himself. It is as if the chains which already exist for the individual between his concepts and words push him in particular directions once the words have been said. For example, which is the odd one out? Pub, house, church, whisky, vat. The answer depends on one's previous experience and on the order in which the words are given.

By a similar token a person can be primed to solve particular problems by being given a list of verbal concepts beforehand; or of course can be primed to make foolish errors. A much quoted example of this is: 'if FOLK is pronounced FOKE, and POLK is pronounced POKE, then how do you pronounce the word which describes the white of an egg?' Many people respond to this in the natural way with the word YOLK (pronounced YOKE) although, of course, the correct answer is ALBUMEN, since it is the *white* of the egg they have been asked for. Or, for example, if red houses are built of red bricks and yellow houses of yellow bricks, what are green houses built of? (Glass, of course.) Priming by certain word chains pushes us in certain directions.

The other important aspect of the role of verbal processes in thinking involves what is termed *linguistic relativity*; this is primarily concerned with differences in language structure between different peoples. This idea began with Whorf's (1940) fascinating hypothesis that a person's perceptions and categorisations (and hence, thoughts) of the world are partially determined by the structure of the language he uses. That is, because his language is structured as it is, it gives him a completely different view of the world from that of someone whose language has a different structure. The sort of example given in support of this hypothesis is that the Hopi Indians in North America have a world view very different from ours because the verb structure of their language is not based on time. It has no past or future tenses, leaving its speakers oriented very much to the present. Or, it is said that the Eskimaux can recognise many more types of snow than we can because they have more words for it. Or, it is said that the Arabs have approximately 6,000 words for camels. Or, to come nearer home, there is the difficulty that English speakers have in recognising colours for which they do not have an appropriate name.

Interesting though the notion of linguistic relativity is, it has not proven to be especially useful or productive, mainly because it is impossible to test directly. Does language shape thought, or thought and world views shape a language? This is an historical question which cannot be answered. In many ways, it might be argued that the similarities between languages and thought processes throughout the world are more impressive than the differences. It may be that language shapes thought to some extent, but it would seem unlikely that it determines a person's overall conception of reality.

Concept Learning

Occasionally in this discussion the word concept has been used; it is now appropriate to say what is meant by this since concept learning, or concept formation, or concept attainment as it is variously called, is a significant aspect of thinking. Clearly, muscular movement, mental images and verbal processes may be involved in thought or at least are corollaries of it; however, also involved, perhaps serving a linking function, are concepts. The basic questions which have been asked here are: how do people form concepts? and what influences the formation of concepts?

Concepts can be defined as: units of knowledge based on experience and involving generalisations into classes of things; or: learned responses (sometimes mental) to common properties found in a variety of stimuli. Basically, concern rests on how a child comes to be able, for example, to label certain moving objects with four wheels as cars rather than as ice-cream floats, prams, skates or even people. Or how he learns to be accurate in distinguishing dogs from other furry four-legged animals. Or how an adult might, for example, learn the correct identification of instances of the style of a particular newspaper.

From these everyday examples it can be seen that the formation of concepts involves both *generalisation* and *discrimination* and probably *selective reinforcement* as well. Consider what happens when a young child is learning the two concepts 'man' and 'Daddy'. At first there is a tentative identification followed rapidly by massive overgeneralisation. He might call all men 'Daddy'; he might call all people 'man'. After this there is a gradual narrowing down. Fewer and fewer men are called 'Daddy', those that have features more and more similar to the child's actual father. Similarly with 'man'. The child gradually learns to put together all the defining features of 'man' versus 'woman' and to apply the labels more accurately (although changes in appearance have made this particular concept more difficult for children today than it was for children 20 or 30 years ago). Generalisations and discrimination seem to be made in the usual way, perhaps aided by selective reinforcement. The child is told by adults when he is right or wrong.

Arguably, the greatest impetus was given to research into concept formation by the work of Bruner, Goodnow and Austin (1956) who carried out a large number of studies in the laboratory. These involved sets of cards on which were simple symbols such as triangles or squares which could vary along a number of dimensions (size, colour, shape, number of borders, etc). The experimenters would say to a subject that they had in mind a particular concept (say, small green circles, or anything not red) and ask him to try to determine what it was by asking whether or not it was embodied in whatever card or cards he chose to indicate. By keeping careful records of choices and by asking questions of the subjects, Bruner, Goodnow and Austin could begin to find out what strategies people use in forming concepts. Of course, it is possible to make the usual criticisms that such a procedure is very artificial in comparison with what occurs in real life, but the chances are that the artificiality would make less difference in this situation than in many others.

From this and similar work it is possible to draw a number of conclusions.

(1) Some concepts are acquired very slowly and others very fast, but all depend on increasing *experiences* with positive and negative instances of the concept. The more experience a person has with furry creatures the better he will become at distinguishing dogs from cats – in our culture.

(2) *Abstraction* and *generalisation* are crucial to concept learning. This means that concept learning always depends on looking at an object or situation and abstracting its essential features (colour, size, shape; hair length, height, depth of voice, etc.). In turn this will depend on previous experiences. So, objects begin to be perceived as similar in some ways; they have essential features in common. These objects would therefore be placed in the same category (people rather than not-

people; telephones rather than not-telephones, etc.). Following the initial processes of abstraction and categorisation, there is generalisation (all objects with certain shared features *must* be telephones) and the generalisations are confirmed or disconfirmed. Whether or not the abstractions and generalisations are done well and appropriately, the two processes always occur in this order.

(3) We appear to categorise in order to *avoid being overwhelmed by discriminations*. If every object a person perceived was in its own individual category he would be placed in an impossible situation in life. Even the most mundane conversation or indeed any bit of behaviour would become impossibly difficult and confusing. In ordinary living, it helps to place objects into identifiable classes. It would be impossible to cut a loaf of bread unless we had built in a category or class of loaves of bread. Otherwise each loaf would be a new experience which would have to be laboriously learned as a basic necessity of life. Categorisation reduces the need for constant learning, it makes action more direct and it allows us to impose some order and structure onto the world and thus to live in it more easily.

(4) In forming concepts we *test hypotheses*. A person makes abstractions and categorisations and then (figuratively) points to what he judges to be instances of the concept, and asks for confirmation. In doing this he learns better from positive than from negative instances, at least in most conditions. In general he learns faster by being told that this *is* an instance of some concept rather than it is not. However, under certain conditions which are not worth exploring here, a negative instance will give more information than a positive instance.

(5) The form of the hypotheses made in concept learning tends to be regular enough to suggest certain general *strategies*. Of these, two main types have been distinguished. The *holistic* strategy begins by being very non-selective and broad and then, as might be expected from its name, develops ponderously but systematically. By contrast, the *partist* strategy begins by dwelling on only one or two aspects of the possible concept and proceeds very inefficiently and haphazardly. It is a good strategy for excluding incorrect hypotheses but unfortunately being so selective it also excludes some elements of what is correct.

(6) Finally, there has been some speculation as to the form which concepts take. It is clear from the discussion in the last section that they can be made up of words or other linguistic symbols. But it is equally clear that this is not a necessary condition. Animals *appear* to be able to form concepts, as can children before they have learned to talk. For example, using operant apparatus and appropriate experimental con-

trols and discrimination procedures, it is possible to train a pigeon to respond only to triangles when it has the choice between these and other shapes. If this continues reliably, it seems reasonable to infer that the pigeon has learned the concept of triangularity. Concept learning in children will not be pursued any further here since children's cognitions will be dealt with in Chapter 14.

Types of Thinking

In this chapter so far, interest has centred only on what might be termed rational thinking — thinking, whether or not it involves language and concept formation, which is towards a particular goal and which follows a fairly logical progression. This type of thinking culminates in reasoning; to which psychologists have given considerable attention. However, before dealing with research into reasoning, it must be pointed out that there are at least four other types of thinking which occur commonly enough to be classed separately. Three of these — free association, fantasy, and delusion can be dealt with quickly. The fourth — creative thinking — is far more important and will be accorded a section to itself.

Free Association

This is a term which is used to apply to thinking which seems to be free both of external cues and from self-instruction. For example, it is something apart from thinking about cars because yours has a rusted exhaust, or thinking about your plans for next week because you judge it best to do so. Rather, it is a succession of thoughts which *appear* to occur in a random sequence, although in fact there is good reason to suppose that each one acts as a stimulus for the next.

Free-association is one of the basic techniques of psychoanalysis. It is believed that the particular sequence of thoughts that occur in free-association, the order in which they occur, and the time gaps between them give clues to a person's innermost desires and wishes, to his unconscious motivation. Take a very obvious example. If a person were to be asked to free-associate to the word 'chair' and his associations were: 'table, kitchen, food, plate, knife, father, kill' and then started off with 'white', he produced: 'black, colour, prejudice, person, child, father, kill'. It would be reasonable to assume that something was wrong in his family relationships.

Fantasies

These are thoughts which are concerned with goals that are unobtainable in real life; castles in the air. Fantasy is a word which often has negative connotations. One thinks of lurid sexual fantasies, or unpleasant fantasies about power, money, or prestige, or of what an individual would like to do to a person whom he envies. However, it is entirely possible, although not proven, that such fantasies may serve the useful function of allowing a person to vent his feelings without much endangering himself or others. Also fantasies can have a direct, positive nature, frequently preceding important creative thoughts for example.

Delusions

These are simply thoughts that revolve around false beliefs. They are irrational thoughts which have particular significance for the individual. They can be about almost anything but usually centre on mistaken notions of *persecution* (the world, or people, or alien beings are out to get you) or *grandeur* (you are Napoleon, or God). They are one of the defining characteristics of the mental disorder known as paranoia, although in limited form they are doubtless experienced by everyone.

Creative Thinking

Creativity is a very difficult topic of study and not one with which psychologists have done particularly well in coming to grips. One reason for this is that much emphasis has been placed on attempts to analyse the creative process itself. What actually happens when an artist paints a picture, a poet creates a poem, a mathematician solves a problem, or a housewife finds a new and better way of coping with the housework? Fascinating questions but extraordinarily difficult to answer since creative thought is such a private matter.

It is possible to ask people questions about creative moments but such a procedure suffers from obvious limitations. If the questions are asked *after* the event then any sort of forgetting may have occurred. If the questions are asked at the time, then they may interfere with the process. However, this is the only way which has been devised to get at creative thinking.

Beginning with Wallas in 1926 there have been several investigators who have attempted to analyse the creative process in scientists and artists. In spite of the crudeness of their methods, results have been surprisingly consistent. They have pointed to four stages in creative thought. At least, they were thought of as stages to begin with, but now they are seen as four aspects of the overall process.

Aspects of creative thinking

(1) Preparation. Essentially, this is scene setting, when the problem is identified and facts gathered which might be pertinent to it.

(2) Incubation. This is perhaps the oddest aspect of creative thinking and involves a time of *no* obvious activity. It is as if no conscious effort at all is being put into the problem; it seems to be constantly ignored.

(3) Illumination. At this point comes the sudden appearance of the creative idea: an 'Aha' experience which seems to occur at unpredictable times and also seems very much like insight. There is a sudden re-seeing or re-evaluation of the problem which heralds a possible solution.

(4) Verification. This includes the evaluation, testing and revision of the ideas produced at the moment of illumination, and is perhaps best seen as the rounding off of the creative process. It involves logical thought and controlled observations and may even end in the rejection of the new ideas.

Although these four aspects of creative thinking have been so often described, they do not provide an adequate model of the processes involved and certainly do not allow much in the way of understanding. There are two main reasons for this. First, the four facets of creativity are no more than descriptions which, although often reported, are not *always* applicable. They cannot therefore be used with any confidence to make predictions. Second, they have little to say about what *exactly* is involved in the moment of illumination or insight, which is of course the time when the creative breakthrough is actually made. Or, by the same token, they have nothing to offer about why the period of so-called incubation is important and what might be happening during it.

Characteristics of Creative Persons

Apart from a burgeoning literature on how to measure creativity, which need not be of concern here, and some work on the possibility of training creativity, the other major emphasis in research has been to take people who are generally regarded to be creative and to see what, if anything, they have in common. Some of the better contributions have been made by Getzels and Jackson (1962) and Terman (1954). In some large-scale studies these investigators found that creative people do indeed share certain characteristics, although it should be said that the results in this field have not always been endorsed; there are many exceptions to the rules.

The main characteristics are:

(1) Individualism − independence of thought and action.

(2) Keen sense of humour.

(3) Given a choice, a strong interest in the novel and the complex rather than the old and simple.

(4) A tolerance of ambiguity.

(5) Perseverance and capacity to work hard.

(6) Self-confidence.

(7) What might be termed bohemianism; a disregard for the conventional.

It is pointless to extend this list any further since it would start to show a lack of consistency. Other investigations have produced other characteristics but they do not hold up well across studies. Also, even if those with proven capacities for creative thought do share some personality characteristics, this still leaves important questions unanswered, as is always the case with findings based simply on correlations. Does the personality lead to the creativity, the creative capacity produce the particular personality, or is there some underlying factor which promotes both the personality and the capacity for creative thought?

Reasoning

Reasoning can be defined as using past experience to solve a current problem, with some likelihood that the individual has derived a principle which can be used in more than one situation. As with other aspects of thinking there is no means of making direct observations of reasoning, so problems have to be devised which, if solved, give good grounds to infer that principles have been worked out and reasoning has occurred.

Given this difficulty in studying reasoning, a basic question which has concerned some psychologists is whether or not animals can reason. A similar question has been asked about young children, but as will be seen in Chapter 14 it has been established beyond doubt that they can. The *double alternation* problem exemplifies the type of situation which has been used with animals. It involves a hungry animal being placed on a number of occasions in a simple T-maze. The difficulty comes in the sequence of turns the animal must make before it finds food, all such turns being made at the same choice point, i.e. where the two segments of the T meet. If for example, it turns right on the first trial, on the next three trials it must turn right, left and left, in that order, i.e. it must learn to make a double alternation.

Rats have great difficulty in learning a double alternation whereas racoons and monkeys can do so more easily. This, and similar evidence, shows that reasoning in animals depends on the complexity of the task, the phylogenetic level of the animals and to some extent on the manner in which the task is fitted to the animal's typical environment.

Enough of animals; they cannot tell us a great deal about human reasoning. It is probably fair to say that there is much of human day-to-day life that requires *no* reasoning at all. On an ordinary working day, getting out of bed, washing, having breakfast and driving to work may all require effort but they are done without reasoning. There are no problems to solve, only well-engrained habits to follow. However, if the car crashes on the way to work and the person wakes up in hospital with a broken leg, then habit is no longer sufficient. He is unexpectedly faced with a large number of problems to solve and he must use his reasoning power. In general, *when habit fails*, reasoning must take over.

Reasoning does not only occur because of the passive failure of habit. Man has curiosity, even though it is very difficult to say whether this is built-in or learned. Certainly, if it is built-in, it is modifiable, since there are many adults who apparently lose some if not all of their share. Nevertheless, to be curious seems to be an important part of being human. And the satisfaction of curiosity requires reasoning.

There are four aspects of reasoning which seem to be more important than others; these again reflect the types of process which occur in many types of thinking.

(1) *Hypotheses.* If a person is given a problem to solve, typically he will generate hypotheses about it. These are possible solutions based on his recall of whatever past experiences seem to be relevant. In general, the more facts he has available, then the greater number of hypotheses he will generate and the better (more likely to lead to solutions) they will be. Also, although it may seem obvious, it is important that the available facts are *relevant*. Take the example of a car stalling; this is very clearly a practical problem which needs solution. If the driver has never before had an engine stall and if he is unfamiliar with the workings of an engine, he can generate very few hypotheses that will help him, and will probably solve his problem by walking to a garage and buying some assistance. If the driver is a mechanic who has owned and worked on many cars most of which have stalled at some time, he will have a variety of facts to draw on which will lead him to generate a neat series of hypotheses based on potential likelihood; and he will soon have solved the problem. These are two obvious examples. But what about the driver who knows nothing of engines but who has experienced

stalling once or twice before? On those occasions he could gain no help but on trying to start the car after ten minutes or so found that it was back to normal. This may leave him with one simple hypothesis based on time. Whatever the trouble is, he thinks that leaving the car for a few minutes will sort it out. He may simply have run out of petrol, a problem which all manner of waiting will not solve. His 'facts' are not relevant to the problem.

(2) Testing. Once generated, hypotheses have to be tested. This is an obvious aspect of reasoning about which little need be said, other than that hypotheses can be tested either empirically (actually tried out) or by more logical thought (if they fall down through being inconsistent with the facts, then they must be wrong, unless the facts are wrong). Also, it is usually best, just as it is in scientific research, to test them one at a time. If two or more are tested together, it is difficult to know which is correct and which is not.

(3) Flexibility. This is the area in which reasoning and creativity come together. Flexibility (with originality and sensitivity) is usually regarded as one of the major facets of creativity. And flexibility is needed in reasoning for the generation of new hypotheses to be tested. A person has assembled all the facts that seem relevant to his problem and none of the hypotheses they have led to produce a solution. It is then that he needs the flexibility to look at the facts in a new way, to generate a fresh hypothesis or even to go back to the problem and find relevant facts that he had forgotten.

Imagine six wine glasses, three full and three empty, arranged in the order FFFEEE and the instruction to move only one of them to produce the order FEFEFE. To solve this problem, you need the flexibility to realise that 'move' need not only mean 'shift' but can also incorporate 'tip'. So you take F*F*F and pour its contents into E*E*E and you have FEFEFE.

(4) Cognition. This final aspect of reasoning harks back to the discussion of transfer of training in Chapter 4, and can be quickly dealt with. It is clear, as in the case of the stalled engine, that prior experience with similar problems is important to the solution of current problems. This can either be seen as a way of knowing more relevant facts and hence generating more and better hypotheses or, if the previous experience is intensive, a way in which habit may take over from reasoning. Similar problems have been met and solved so often before that

familiar chains of behaviour are quickly worked through. Compare for instance the earlier example of the man who wakes up (for the first time) in hospital with a broken leg, with the jockey who is taken to hospital for the twentieth time with a broken collar bone. On the face of it they have similar problems, but in the case of the jockey the problem and its solution are so familiar that he will barely have to think about it.

Faulty Reasoning

The above discussion has proceeded largely on the basis that reasoning occurs with some clarity and follows perfect logical progressions. Naturally, this is not always so. Reasoning is often faulty. This may not just be due to having only a few relevant facts or inappropriate previous experiences, but can also occur for at least three other reasons.

(1) Inappropriate set. Each of us, unless abnormally flexible, brings a set way of responding to bear on any problem, and being in a set pattern is the opposite of being flexible. Sometimes the set may be appropriate to the problem, but sometimes not; when it is inappropriate it can lead to faulty reasoning. Take the person who starts to have dizzy spells and frequent headaches. These are inconvenient and painful so he is concerned and begins to speculate about the causes. His father died from a brain tumour so this 'sets' him to find that particular solution. He convinces himself and becomes more and more worried. The reasoning is faulty because he has not generated and tested other possible (and simpler) hypotheses. In fact his vision is defective, and if corrected with glasses his headaches and dizziness would disappear.

(2) A second way in which reasoning might be faulty is through *functional fixedness.* This again is a way of being inflexible in thinking and is a matter of seeing objects as only capable of functioning in their usual way. Pens, for example, can be used in many ways other than simply for writing. Recently, I heard of a couple whose car had broken down miles from anywhere when they were on a picnic. They had no tools and little expertise, but it was obvious that the trouble was caused by a severed wire. They joined the wire together with foil taken from their wine bottle and tied this in place with the stretched plastic skin from a sausage. It was enough to get them to a garage. Seeing the wine bottle as only a wine bottle and a sausage only as a sausage would have prevented this solution.

(3) *Faulty logic* usually shows up in what is termed *syllogistic* reasoning. A syllogism is a three part statement, the third part following

from the premises of the first two. Thus for example, A is greater than B, B is greater than C; it follows that A is greater than C. When the logic is faulty in this context it takes the form of drawing a conclusion which does not follow from the first two statements.

For example: I am fat and want to reduce weight. Diets reduce weight. It follows that to reduce weight I must diet. Although this *may* be true it does not follow logically. The person might be fat due to some metabolic disturbance that is unmalleable by diet. Also, diets are not the only way to reduce weight; exercise might be more appropriate in this case. Examples of logic as faulty as this abound in everyday life. Take a final instance: I want to pass my examinations but have not done enough work. People who work hard read a great deal. If I read a lot I will pass my examinations. Unfortunately, this follows neither in logic nor in practice, necessarily.

Theories of Thinking

As is the case when considering any of the higher mental processes such as memory or thinking there are two main types of theory. One comes from the tradition of learning theory and stimulus-response psychology, and the other is purely cognitive.

Stimulus-response theory views thinking as explicable by an extension of the principles of learning, more particularly as a matter of the formation of stimulus-response connections (S-R). For the most part, in learning theory itself stimuli and responses are overt and observable, but this cannot be the case with thinking. Of course, thought processes may begin with external stimuli and may end with full-blown muscular responses, but learning theorists would argue that lesser stimuli and responses (s–r) mediate between these. Thus, an external stimulus activates cognitive processes which are usually described as symbolic. These processes themselves can react on one another by chains of small stimuli and responses. So the lesser s's and r's act as mediating or intervening links until eventually the big R, or overt response results.

In simple diagrammatic form, the learning theory account of thinking is: S-- (s-r-s-rs-r . . .) --R. Although the mediating s-r connections are entirely hypothetical, some theorists argue that they have a potential physical substrate in the neural processes of the brain. From this viewpoint they are really neuronal linkages. However, such a view has not been proven and at present is difficult to test.

Cognitive theorists of thinking regard the S-R view as over-simplified. The main reason for this is that they feel it entirely unjustified to leave out the activity of the organism. So they are S-O-R theorists rather than S-R theorists. The reason they argue in this way is that they feel the proof to be incontrovertible that thinking involves processes such as understanding, hypothesis testing and problem solving. This seems very different from the rather simple formation and then checking of stimulus-response connections.

The cognitive theorist regards thinking as an *active* rather than a passive process, concerned with the utilisation of signs, symbols and other internal representations of the world. He sees thinking as involving a hierarchical arrangement of superordinate and subordinate ideas. Linkages in the thought process are formed instantaneously and the thinker has to go through the various possibilities and test which is correct. Although this is an active process, it will be constrained by the hierarchical arrangements which already exist in his cognitions.

This is sufficient to give the flavour of the two types of theory of thinking. They are interesting because they are based essentially on one set of facts and simply represent two very different ways of interpreting them. S-R theory has the advantages of simplicity and derivations from other well-tried areas, and the possible disadvantages of over-simplification and viewing thinking as rather passive. Cognitive theory has the advantages of considering the person as a complex cognitive being and thinking as an active process, and the possible disadvantages of being very difficult to test convincingly. The main problem for any theory of thinking is that which would apply to a theory of any type of *mental* process. That is, the difficulty of bringing the gap between this and the body within which, or as part of which, it occurs.

Abnormalities in Thinking

As a final brief discussion in this chapter it is worth spending a few lines on possible abnormalities in thinking. Some of these are mentioned in other chapters and there has already been discussion above of the delusional thoughts which typify conditions such as paranoia. In general, neurotics do not show very much impairment in their thinking or intellectual abilities. On the other hand, there seems to be progressive impairment and distortions of thinking in psychotic conditions such as schizophrenia and the affective disorders. However, if and when the patient recovers, his thought processes systematically return to normal.

To mention a few more specific problems:
(1) Schizophrenics are particularly poor on abstract reasoning.
(2) Extroverts are more careless and impulsive in their thinking than are others.

(3) Psychotics make more errors in thinking than non-psychotics.

(4) Strong feelings of depression and guilt often lead to high distractibility through a lack of concentration.

(5) Anxiety reduces memory span and hence impairs thinking.

(6) Older people cannot learn as well as younger people, their apparent problems with memory and thinking really being difficulties with learning.

(7) Schizophrenics have difficulty in forming new concepts, although those they do form tend to be unusual.

(8) Schizophrenics sometimes tend to include too many (inappropriate) items in the concepts they form, which, in itself, could account for their cognitive difficulties.

Overall, either extreme mental disorder or extreme age does seem to lead to impairment in thinking, sometimes directly and sometimes indirectly through effects on memory and learning. The main types of disability are slowness, loss of reasoning power, and distractibility. Such effects can also result from short term problems such as illness and injury or other stresses, and from more transient states such as having consumed too much alcohol.

Summary Points

(1) Thinking is a process involving the manipulation of ideas and images; mental representations of the external world. It usually progresses by defining a problem, sorting out related concepts, and forming and testing hypotheses.

(2) There are various correlates of thinking – such as muscle activity – although these are not necessary to thinking.

(3) One of the major mediators of thinking is language, although again language is not necessary to thinking. There is some debate over whether language is shaped by thought or thought shaped by language.

(4) A particular form of thinking is concept learning or formation which is the classification of objects into various categories according to their points of similarity and difference. Crucial to concept formation are abstraction, generalisation, discrimination, and probably selective reinforcement. It appears that we form concepts in order to avoid being overwhelmed by discriminations and in so doing form and test hypotheses. The two main strategies in concept formation are holistic and partist.

(5) Apart from concept learning and reasoning, the main types of thinking are free-association, fantasy, delusion, and creativity.

(6) Creativity is difficult to study but such research as there is suggest that it has four aspects: preparation, incubation, illumination and verification. There is some evidence that creative persons share certain personality characteristics such as independence and a liking for the novel and complex.

(7) Reasoning has to take over when habit fails. It usually involves four processes: formation of hypotheses, testing of hypotheses, flexibility, and cognition. Faulty reasoning may be due to: inappropriate sets, functional fixedness, or faulty logic.

(8) The two major explanations of thinking are in terms of the stimulus-response connections of learning theory or the more active hypothesis-testing approach of cognitive psychology.

(9) There are various conditions which can lead to deteriorations or distortions in thinking. They are usually dependent on extreme mental disorder or old age, although they may also result from more short-lived conditions.

Study Questions – 7

(1) List the instances of faulty thinking you have seen during your training. Do they fit into systematic categories? Has your own training led you to think in particular ways?

(2) Assess the abilities of your patients to solve problems. How would you vary your approach according to the type of error a patient has made?

(3) Collect examples of faulty reasoning on the part of your patients. Do you think that these are different within a hospital than in the outside world?

(4) From what you have seen in your training and in your work, do people think actively or passively? What are the differences between the two?

(5) Does it appear to you that some people think more than others? Why? What is happening when people are apparently *not* thinking? What experiences might lead your patients to give this appearance?

(6) Does it appear to you that some of your patients and your colleagues can concentrate better and persevere longer than others? Why do you think that this should be so? What is different about such people?

(7) Do you believe it to be possible to tell what people are thinking simply by watching them? If so, how? If not, why not?

(8) Test the capacities of your patients to form concepts, particularly

about the hospital and the treatment you are giving them, where this is possible. Do they differ in their capacities to do this?

(9) What aspects of your training have led you to think creatively? What happens when you do so? Do you think that the setting in which you work promotes or inhibits creative thinking?

(10) During the course of your studies and your work have you seen any types of thinking not mentioned in this chapter? What are they and how have they come about?

8 EMOTION

Definitions and Problems of Study

Although emotion is such a common aspect of everyday experience, from the psychologist's viewpoint it stands out as a word which is extremely difficult to define. This is so much the case that some psychologists have advocated doing away with the term altogether. Try a simple exercise. Think for a moment or two about emotion and try to say to yourself what it is. Write down a definition.

If you have done this, then you will almost certainly have covered some, if not all, of the following points.

(1) Emotion involves *feeling*, personal subjective experience. All of us know of situations in which someone has made us feel happy or sad or angry or jealous, and so on. Sometimes such feelings seem to be overwhelming and to last for hours or even days. At other times they are short-lived but intense. And at others they are brief momentary flashes, very mild in nature of which we may not even be able to trace the cause. They are part of everyday life, qualifying general behaviour and sometimes seriously interfering with it.

(2) Emotion involves *behaviour*. It is possible to see emotion in action. If a person is angry he may tremble or fight; if a person is sad he hangs his head, hunches his shoulders and seems to have no energy for life.

(3) Linked to the obvious behavioural signs of emotion are its equally important *physiological* facets. An angry person becomes red (or white) in the face; he sweats; he can feel his heart pumping faster and his respiration rate increases. Adrenalin is coursing round his body preparing him for action.

(4) Finally, in defining emotion you probably made mention of the *situation* which provoked it. All emotion occurs in response to some stimulus, which is usually social. A member of a person's family speaks in a particular way and this arouses emotion in him.

Because emotion involves each of these four aspects, there has been some confusion in the way in which it has been studied. Typically, investigators have chosen to emphasise one or other of these facets of emotion at the expense of the others, and to construct theories and carry out research which reflects whatever their biasses might be. A further complexity is apparent if one considers that these various facets of emotion might occur separately rather than together, and hence have

130

complex influences on one another. Is it necessary to study the subjective side of emotion at all? Does it have a causative role to play in
emotion or is it merely something which goes along in parallel to emotional behaviour and physiological responses?

This is but one of many problems with which the study of emotion
abounds. It is worth mentioning a few of these at this stage since they
should be borne in mind throughout the remainder of this chapter.
(1) In studying emotion, ideally one would like to know what another
person is feeling. How is this possible? The only information available
comes from the person's facial expression and bodily reactions, knowledge of whatever led up to his responses, and a projection of what one
would be feeling if in a similar situation.
(2) People react quite differently to the same emotional stimulus. A
social slight may go unnoticed by one person, be reacted to with anger
by the next, and might make a third anxious. One person might become
angry and aggressive with the mildest of goads whilst the next remains
phlegmatic under the most intense provocation. This problem means
that specific emotions as they are known in everyday life have not
received very much study by psychologists, although anxiety and anger
are exceptions to this.
(3) Given the complexity of emotion, is it possible to study it scientifically? The study of emotion highlights the dilemma which exists between real-life investigations and their relative lack of control, as contrasted with the greater control but obvious artificiality of laboratory
investigation. Some would argue that it is impossible to study emotion
in the laboratory at all realistically. As soon as the individual knows he
is in an artificial situation then his emotional reactions will be tempered
or qualified in some way.

For example, how would it be possible to make someone genuinely
angry in a laboratory? His anger, if it could be aroused at all (and there
would of course be ethical objections made even to the attempt) would
probably be quite different from that in everyday life. And even if it
were not, how could the investigator be sure whether it was or not, or
even make some guess as to the extent of the similarity?
(4) The complexity of emotion is also reflected in problems of measurement. Assume that the above problems have been overcome and that a
person has been made angry or anxious or whatever; how would this be
measured? Would one measure his behaviour, his physiological
responses, his feelings, the effects of his emotion on some task he had
been set, or what?
(5) One type of solution to all these problems, including ethical ones, is

to use animals in the study of emotion. This of course brings problems of a different order. How do we know that animals have emotions at all? It is possible to see them respond in apparently emotional ways, and dog lovers have no doubts at all. But this is not objective enough. How could we ever know what an animal feels? It may not be that animals experience emotions in the same way as humans, and even if they do, it may not be that the same processes underlie their emotions as underlie ours.

Even if it is assumed that the study of animal emotion may give useful pointers to an understanding of human emotion, it is possible to study only a very limited range of emotions in this way. It would be difficult to make an animal elated, or guilty, or depressed.

(6) A final problem concerns the words of emotion. These are very familiar in everyday life. People speak confidently of happiness, anger, sadness, jealousy, and so on. But as soon as one tries to define such words they become very hard to pin down; they carry a great deal of surplus meaning. This problem is compounded by the way in which people learn to name emotions. Our parents see us in particular situations, project themselves into the situation and then speak to us of them. 'Don't be angry', 'If you do that you'll only be fed up in the end', 'What have you got that long face about?' It is through these comments and questions that we come to label what we feel in various situations.

A learning process such as this will be slightly different for everyone. Since subjective feelings and complex social situations are involved, it is a very different matter from learning to label concrete objects such as tables and chairs. Each person's experiences will be unique and his understanding of the terms of emotion will also be unique. In studying emotion, the psychologist has to try to find ways of putting aside these unique, idiosyncratic aspects and get at essential meanings in order to make meaningful generalisations. This can be very difficult.

Early Theories of Emotion

For many centuries in the writings of philosophers, emotion was contrasted with reason, emotion being seen as base and animal-like and reason being seen as good and particularly human. This contrast persists in society today and still provides one of the rules of life. Be rational; do not be governed by your emotions.

However, this theory has never been productive of research or of improving an understanding of emotion. Towards the end of the last century theories of emotion became more psychological in their expression, the first of them taking the simple form of: stimulus-emotion-response. Then William James reversed this view with what has become the very influential James-Lange theory of emotion (1884). He suggested that if someone calls you a liar, for example, you might strike him and *then* feel angry. It is the feedback from the act of striking and from the aroused internal state that produces the anger. The importance of this theory was that it emphasised the significance of bodily states to emotion. Although this may seem obvious now it was James who made it so.

The theory which is usually contrasted with that of James is Cannon's who carried out much of his work in the 1920s. He argued that emotion is mediated particularly in the thalamic areas of the brain. External stimuli are picked up by receptors which relay impulses to the cortex. This in turn excites thalamic processes which act in patterns corresponding to particular emotional expression. Thalamic discharge both excites muscles and viscera and also relays information back to the cortex.

Cannon also emphasised the functions of the autonomic nervous system in preparing the individual for fight or flight. The parasympathetic division serves for bodily conservation. Then, in times of stress, the stored energy is made rapidly available for whatever emotional course of action is appropriate. Cannon's theory then was essentially physiological, laying great stress on the adaptive nature of emotional reactions.

In the early part of this century there was much discussion as to the relative merits of these two theories. More recently this has died down a little and has been replaced by a considerable divergence of viewpoints. Some psychologists have promoted the importance of physiological change, others have concentrated on behaviour, and others have dwelt on the cognitive aspects of emotion. Sometimes a theorist has even combined two or more of these aspects. Since research has also followed these broad divisions they will be used in the following discussion.

Physiology and Emotion
It is absolutely self-evident that physiological change is implicated in emotion. Since James onwards, hundreds of experiments have shown that general emotionality is related to the working of the autonomic nervous system, particularly in fear, rage, and intense excitement. The general changes which take place in these conditions are that all functions of the gastro-intestinal system are stopped or slowed down, the heart beats faster and more blood is circulated to the musculature than to the gut. These effects are enhanced by the secretion of adrenalin

which promotes more sympathetic discharge, hence prolonging the emotional excitement.

These physiological changes are usually measured indirectly by polygraphic recordings made at the periphery via electrodes placed on the surface of the body to measure, for example, skin resistance, heart rate, rate of respiration, muscle tones, and so on. As such they form the basis of the lie detector, which is based on the idea that although a person might be able to control the overt behaviour involved in what he does or says, his physiological responses will sometimes give him away.

There are various physiological theories of emotion, Arnold (e.g. 1960) having a great deal to say in her comprehensive work on the subject. However, although these point very clearly to certain areas of the brain being especially implicated in emotion (the brain stem, the hypothalamus, the thalamus, the limbic system, and, to a limited extent, the neocortex), the theories themselves remain at the speculative level when it comes to fine detail. They will not be considered any further.

More important from the physiological viewpoint is the question of whether or not there is any evidence for *physiological response patterning* in emotion. Since James pointed to the importance of the viscera the search has been on for patterns of physiological responses which differentiate the various emotions. The idea of such patterns would seem reasonable since from the subjective viewpoint, emotions *seem* to be quite distinct from one another.

Of the many studies carried out in this search, it is very few which have offered positive evidence. Probably the most famous is that of Wolf and Wolff (1943) who were able to study the reactions of a man's stomach (he had a gastric fistula) to stimuli which would normally provoke fear and those which would normally provoke rage. They found that fear reduced gastric activity and blood flow and that anger produced a different pattern. However, more recent studies have been by no means as clear cut in their results as was this one.

Although one might expect there to be obvious patterns to the various emotions this seems simply *not* to be so. Of overriding importance is the fact that an individual appears to have typical patterns of general emotional response, but that such patterns vary considerably from person to person. Even the differences between fear and anger do not show up well between studies and between individuals.

Cognition and Emotion

Research and theory into cognitive involvement in emotion has recently been more illuminating and influential than that which stresses physiology alone. This has been due largely to the work of Schachter (e.g. 1971) which will be described in some detail. The impetus for his work came from a study conducted many years ago in which the investigator injected some 200 subjects with adrenalin and then asked them to describe what it made them feel. About 70 per cent of them reported that it made them feel *as if* they were afraid, rather than making them feel afraid directly. The injections produced 'as if' reactions, putting them in an emotional state for which they could find no good explanation.

This led Schachter to put forward three propositions, which he subsequently bore out in a series of experimental investigations. The propositions were based on the belief that emotion comes about through a mixture of stimuli from outside and from feelings and thoughts from inside.
(1) If we are emotionally aroused and there seems to be no good reason for this, then we will label our emotions with whatever thoughts we may have about what is going on around us at the time.
(2) If we are aroused emotionally and there *is* an obvious reason for it, then we will be satisfied and will not seek for further explanations.
(3) If emotion is to occur at all then we must be aroused, physiologically.

Essentially then Schachter was suggesting that although physiological arousal is necessary to emotion, cognitive factors may be a major determinant of emotional states. Although this idea gave rise to a large series of investigations, ranging from studies of obesity to studies of crime, it is the first which is worth describing in some detail. This was carried out by Schachter and Singer in 1962.

Schachter and Singer duped their subjects into believing that they were studying the effects of an injected vitamin on vision. However, the subjects were in fact injected with either adrenalin or a weak saline solution (which would have no effects – it was simply to control for the effects of giving an injection). The subjective effects of adrenalin injections are palpitations, tremors, flushing, increased respiration, and so on. In Schachter's study these effects lasted for about 20 minutes. The subjects were either told what to expect (as possible side effects of the supposed vitamin injection), were told to expect entirely different and quite impossible side-effects, or were told nothing at all.

After receiving their injections, the experimental subjects were taken individually into another room purportedly to wait for the injection to take effect. Here, they waited with another person whom they believed to be an experimental subject like themselves. This man was in fact a confederate of the experimenters. This bogus subject would then begin to behave in one of two rather bizarre ways. With some individuals he became very euphoric, laughing and joking, messing up the room, and inveigling the real subject into playing various games. With others he became more and more angry whilst they were filling in a questionnaire together, eventually stalking out of the room altogether. Whilst all this was going on the subjects were being watched by hidden observers, their emotional states being assessed. They also had to fill in post-experimental questionnaires about their feelings during the experiment.

The general finding from this complex study was that those subjects who had been injected with adrenalin but had *not* been told what to expect became far more angry or euphoric than the others. They more quickly picked up the emotional states of the confederate subjects. They had been made physiologically aroused but had no explanation for this. So they evaluated what was going on emotionally in their immediate environment and used this to label their state. Other subjects (with explanations or injected with only saline) did not behave in this way. Thus Schachter gained support for his three propositions with one study.

Of course in everyday life the situation is far more complex than was the case in Schachter's study. In any conversation for example there is a constant interplay between what is going on inside a person and his evaluation of what is occurring outside. There is incessant influence and interaction between the two. In mild ways one is constantly being aroused emotionally and is casting around for ways of accounting for this.

Schachter's general findings and beliefs about emotion have had many ramifications, both empirical and theoretical. On the empirical side, for example, Schachter and others have carried out a series of studies on obesity. In general, these studies endorse the idea that obese people are distinguishable from those of normal weight because they eat more in response to external cues such as the sight and smell of food, the time of day, their surroundings and so on, than to internal cues such as their state of physiological hunger. By contrast, people of normal weight place far more importance on their physiological state.

More theoretically, Schachter's ideas suggest that the earlier views that emotions are merely bodily changes are too simplistic. Due recognition must also be given to 'mental' events such as remembering, perceiving, and making judgements. People hold large ranges of expectancies, labels, judgements and memories which combine with the bodily reactions to produce the experienced emotion. Schachter might even argue that the mental events *are* the emotion since he has shown that it is these which make one emotion distinguishable from the next.

Appraisals

In the last section it was mentioned that from the cognitive viewpoint in emotion we make various judgements. These have been more usually termed appraisals and form an important part of the theories of Arnold (1960) and Lazarus (1968). The basic question is that if appraisals are important to emotion, how are they made? Something happens which we appraise as good or bad for us; how do we do it?

The central idea in these theories is that if we appraise something as good then we tend to approach it, and if we appraise it as bad then we tend to avoid it. Of course, few situations are as clear-cut as this. We make multiple appraisals with good and bad elements to them and we constantly re-appraise. Thus, a person perceives something and also immediately appraises it. If this produces a strong tendency to do something about it then emotion is experienced.

Such speculation seems reasonable. We do not feel emotional about everything. My appraisals of a person whom I know, will be far more likely to be emotional than my appraisals of a table. Appraisal theorists such as Arnold argue that appraisals depend on past experiences. If you see somebody or somebody says something to you, this reminds you of similar experiences and revives memories of emotions you felt at the time. These remembered emotions will colour your judgements and make you become anxious or angry or whatever. Also, you will make predictions or guesses. We all do this constantly in social situations. If the conversation continues what form will it take? What will it mean for you? Will he make you angry again? You use your memory and imagination to determine what seems to be the best course of action to follow.

Arnold's theory also goes back to the old dichtomy between emotion and reason. She distinguishes between deliberate action and emotional appraisal. For example, you are out walking, see a rain cloud and take shelter; perception, appraisal, deliberate rational judgements. You are out walking, see someone who made you extremely angry yesterday and cross the street to avoid him, walking very stiffly and with a prickly feeling in your shoulders: perception, appraisal, action, all in terms of emotional consequences.

Lazarus's view of appraisal is slightly different from that of Arnold. He suggests that appraisals can be either benign or threatening. Benign appraisals have three possible adaptive consequences:

(1) There might be adaptive *automatic coping* with no emotion involved. We cross the road and automatically jump out of the way of a bus.

(2) There might be information provided that means that a re-appraisal must be made. A man gazes fondly out of the window at his new car and sees it scratched by someone parking clumsily.

(3) A benign appraisal may lead to a positive emotional state.

Alternatively, threatening appraisals involve two processes.

(1) Evaluation of the threat.

(2) Evaluation of how to cope with the threat

In turn, the first of these may lead to *direct* action, to remove the threat. Feedback from this would clearly be important to emotion. Or it may lead to a *benign re-appraisal*, which is entirely cognitive and is what happens when no direct action seems possible. Again though, any fluctuations in emotion are seen as continuous appraisal and re-appraisal. It should be borne in mind however that although such ideas might seem perfectly reasonable and to make good subjective sense, for the most part they are speculative.

Behaviour and Emotion

Some theorists and researchers have argued that it is unnecessary to consider the cognitive aspects of emotion at all; they do not have a causal role to play but merely go on in parallel to any emotional behaviour which is occurring. They would also argue that it is fruitless to consider physiological responses since these only underlie what is going on at the behavioural level. Therefore, the proper study of emotion should be made at the behavioural level alone; a true behaviourist approach.

This standpoint has its origins in a study which was carried out in 1920 by Watson (the so-called father of behaviourism) and Raynor. They reported a dramatic demonstration of fear conditioning in an eleven-month-old child called Albert. To begin with he was allowed to play with a friendly white rat, which he did quite happily for some time. After this, whenever he reached out for the rat a loud noise would be made behind him. This brought about emotional behaviour — whimpering, hiding his head and so on. After the sight of the rat and the loud noise had been paired together a number of times, the sight of the rat alone would bring out the emotional reactions; a straightforward case of classical conditioning. The learned response generalised to a number of other objects, mainly those which were furry.

Watson argued that this demonstration was simply a parallel to the conditioning of emotion which occurs in real life. He suggested that we are born with three built-in patterns of emotion which occur automatically (unconditioned) to certain stimuli. In his behaviouristic way he termed these X, Y and Z, although they correspond roughly to what others might term fear, rage and love. Thereafter he suggested that all our emotions are conditioned in the way that little Albert's fear was conditioned. And of course the implication is that they could be extinguished as can all learned responses.

These ideas of Watson have led to the development of an approach to the study of emotion which has come to be known as *conditioned emotional responding.* The basic procedure involves the establishment of some on-going operant behaviour at a steady rate. Once this is established, a classical conditioning procedure is superimposed upon it. A neutral stimulus is presented for a brief period of time and is terminated with an even briefer presentation of an unconditioned stimulus which is known to evoke emotional behaviour.

Although this procedure sounds complex, it is in fact quite straightforward. Thinking back to Chapter 2, consider a rat pressing a bar in a Skinner box for food at a steady rate. Whilst he is doing this, occasionally a buzzer sounds for some seconds at the end of which the rat receives an electric shock to his feet. At first the shock leads to a general cessation in bar pressing. Then, as the number of pairings of buzzer and shock increase (pairings of CS and US), the suppression in bar pressing becomes restricted to the time when the buzzer is sounding and recovers again immediately after the shock. This suppression during the CS has come to be known as conditioned anxiety, its extent depending on many variables such as the intensity of the US, the duration of the CS and the type of operant baseline on which the classical conditioning is superimposed.

This general procedure should become clearer with an everyday example, which surprisingly enough is easy to find. Consider a typist who is relatively happy in her work and sits typing at a fairly steady rate during the day. Occasionally her boss of whom she is a little in awe, makes the rounds of his employees. She can always hear him doing this by the sound of him moving along the corridor and going into various rooms. This always lasts for some ten minutes before he eventually arrives at her room. It is reasonable to predict that her work would be in some way disrupted during that ten minutes when she can hear his progress. This is very like superimposing a neutral stimulus (the sound of her boss) linked to a mildly negative stimulus (the boss himself) on a steady rate on positively reinforced (by money) behaviour (typing).

The type of conditioned anxiety is only one of a number of possibilities for studying conditioned emotional responding. The others are shown in the table below. In this table the positive baseline refers to some ongoing operant behaviour which is maintained by positive reinforcement (say food to a hungry animal). The negative baseline refers to some steady operant behaviour which is maintained by negative reinforcement (such as the avoidance of an electric shock, for example). Superimposed on these two types of baseline can be neutral stimuli which precede four types of emotion-provoking stimuli: S- (e.g. electric shock), S+ (e.g. food), $- (e.g. 'time-out' from electric shock), and $+ (e.g. 'time-out' from food). This leads to the six possible situations which are shown in Table 8.1.

Table 8.1: Possible Ways to Study Conditioned Emotional Responding

	CS--S-	CS-S+	CS-$-	CS-$+
Positive baseline	anxiety	elation	—	anger
Negative baseline	anxiety	elation	relief	—

(The two blanks in the table occur because although they are logical possibilities for study they are not practically possible.)

Although these procedures cannot be denied and one can find examples of them in everyday life, many people would argue that they are far removed from emotion, particularly since they have almost always been studied in animals. Is it at all reasonable to label the various cells in the table anxiety, elation, anger, and relief? In dealing with behaviour alone and representing rather complex experimental procedures as they do, they seem to lose much of the richness of emotion as it is experienced. Also of course, they do not dwell on the direct study of emotional reactions. The effect of the conditioned emotion is always seen against a baseline of some on-going behaviour. As far as it goes this is fair, but perhaps it does not go far enough. An understanding of emotion will come not only from seeing the disruptive or enhancing effects it has on other behaviour, but also from an analysis of it in its own right.

Be this as it may, these ideas have led to the development of a theory of emotion which is couched sheerly in behavioural terms (Millenson, 1967). It rests on the basic proposition that emotional changes which occur through classical condtioning, either promote or suppress other, non-emotional behaviour. Millenson suggests that some emotions differ only in intensity and that some emotions are basic whilst others are compounds of these. This, and the sort of analysis made above lead him to a three-dimensional model of emotion which clearly has much in common with Watson's X, Y and Z ideas.

Dimension 1 is terror, anxiety and apprehension which sometimes suppress and sometimes enhance operant behaviour.

Dimension 2 is elation or pleasure which enhances operant behaviour.

Dimension 3 is anger which facilitates some operant behaviour and leads to attack and destruction.

Finally, Millenson argues that more complex emotions develop from mixtures of these three emotions. To take one example, guilt results from pleasure from possessing something which we should not have, and anxiety about being caught.

Anxiety

Although it was said earlier in this chapter that psychologists have not paid much attention to the study of specific emotions, the major exception to this is anxiety, on which an enormous amount of research has been done. For this reason, and also because it exemplifies the study of abnormal emotion it is worth spending some time in its discussion. In reading what follows it should be remembered that it is very difficult to define what is meant by abnormality and particularly what exactly is abnormal anxiety. This is largely a matter of degree, which is always arbitrary, and also an area in which there are considerable individual differences.

The main problem in defining anxiety, although we all know from subjective experiences something of what it is, is that of deciding whether it is better characterised as a convenient *short-hand term* for a group of behaviours or as an *internal state* which causes certain behaviour. The word anxiety has been in use in both ways by various psychologists.

Neurotic Anxiety

The person suffering from general neurotic anxiety breathes very fast, his heart pumps faster than usual and he sweats overmuch. His blood pressure rises and he defecates and urinates often. His mouth feels dry and his skin looks pale. If this condition continues he begins to show signs of nervous irritability, his digestion being impaired and his sleep broken.

Usually the anxious person feels some sort of apprehension or threat which must be dealt with. But he does not know what its cause is or what he should do. It is obviously maladaptive. Such anxiety can come about as a corollary of bodily organic disorders, or of depressive psychoses. It is associated with adolescence and old age. As well as these general factors there are more specific factors which seem to precipitate anxiety. These can occur through any sort of physical or emotional stress. Even given all these conditions some people do not become anxious. As mentioned before there are enormous individual differences involved.

Emotionally, anxiety is a most unpleasant state which often leads to depression. The person is irritable, tired and lacking in concentration. He is frustrated and impatient. To relax he must solve his problems but not only does he not know how to do this, he does not even know what they are. This description is of extremes, which most of us fortunately never experience. On the other hand, all but a very few experience mild anxiety. This seems to be highly appropriate since, all other things being equal, people with a moderate level anxiety, when facing some task, tend to do better at it than those who are extremely anxious, and also than those who are not anxious at all; examinations provide a good example of this.

As well as this general form, neurotic anxiety is also seen in the *phobic reactions* — these are irrational fears which can be of almost anything. One of the most common phobias is agoraphobia, or fear of open spaces. It usually takes the form of a gradually increasing fear of leaving the house until in the end the very *thought* of going out puts the person in an anxious state and he or she becomes completely housebound.

Anxiety is arguably the most common emotion. In mild form we all experience it and it can be useful in acting as a motivator. In more extreme form it can make considerable inroads into vitality, eventually becoming thoroughly debilitating. It is the emotion which provides the basis for the neuroses and as such is strongly associated with depression.

Theories of Anxiety

There have been numerous theories of anxiety, but these can be grouped into various types. In this section three types will be described which exemplify reasonably different approaches to the topic.

All theories of anxiety begin with Freud who has been very influential in this field. He distinguished between *objective* anxiety and *neurotic* anxiety. He described both of these as signals of danger but felt that the former came from the real external world and that the latter came from within. Neurotic anxiety is what is of interest here. Freud described four stages in its development.

(1) A child is punished for an aggressive or sexual impulse.

(2) The child becomes objectively anxious about the possibility of similar punishment in the future.

(3) He attempts to be free of this anxiety by repressing anything which is associated with the antisocial impulses.

(4) Later, this repression breaks down partially and the anxiety surfaces although not attached to anything in the environment. The person is not aware that the repression has occurred in the first place.

According to Freud, this type of anxiety is basic to all the neuroses.

The second type of theory was put forward by Epstein (1967). He based it on an interesting series of comparisons between novice and experienced parachutists. As the time approached for their jump, novices said that they were more anxious, a condition which Epstein confirmed physiologically. However, the peak of anxiety for the experienced parachutists was quite remote from the jump. At first they were not anxious, then as the jump drew nearer their anxiety rose and decreased just as sharply just before the jump. The more their experience, the more remote in time from the jump was the peak of their anxiety.

These results led Epstein to propose a general theory of anxiety and of how people learn to cope with it. He views anxiety as an *undirected state of arousal* which follows the perception of danger. We are aroused but do not know how to act to reduce the unpleasantness. Mastery involves trying to channel the anxiety in some specific direction so that something can actually be done about it. Neurotic anxiety builds up and worsens if it is impossible to do this.

Spielberger's (1966) ideas on anxiety stem from the fact that by and large psychologists have tended to think of anxiety in one of two ways.

(1) They see anxiety as a complex response to events in the world, something that we all experience from time to time. This is characterising anxiety as a *state*, rather like a mood which lasts for a definite and rather short period of time.

(2) Others have viewed anxiety as a personality *trait*, an enduring characteristic which is part of the nature of most people.

Spielberger suggests that these two conceptualisations could be usefully combined to form a *state-trait* idea of anxiety. The fluctuating state of anxiety would have subjective feelings of vague apprehension, threat and tension. And the nervous system would set us up for emergency reactions. A personality trait of anxiety would be like a disposition which makes us more or less ready than the next person to see threats and dangers in the world. States of anxiety depend on the appraisal of a situation as threatening, whereas anxiety as a trait would reflect earlier experiences, perhaps of childhood, which have made us more or less prone to anxiety.

Although this state-trait view of anxiety is well thought out and has much to be said for it, it still carries its problems. For example, is a person who is in a state of extreme general anxiety really in a state, or is he simply showing a complex set of behavioural reactions? Do these reactions stand alone or are they the anxiety? Are they symptomatic of something deeper? Is this normal or abnormal, in general or for the individual?

Causes of Anxiety

It is important to say a final word about two of the ways in which the causes of anxiety have been conceptualised. One suggestion is that abnormal anxiety has its roots in childhood experiences, an idea proposed by Freud but greatly extended by others. The anxiety is thought to develop through the loss to the child of some loved person with whom he has had an affectionate relationship. After this, anxiety will be aroused by any disturbance in social relationships.

The original anxiety is termed *separation anxiety*, which of course anyone would feel. It only becomes abnormal when it is extreme. The more frequent and more extreme are the child's experiences of being separated from his parents or guardians, then the more severe will be his anxiety reactions. As an adult he will be that much more likely to overreact to social upsets.

A second hypothesis concerning the causes of anxiety dwells on possible genetic influences; the potential for anxiety may be inherited. For example, about fifteen per cent of the parents and siblings of anxiety neurotics are also highly anxious. More important, an identical twin with an anxiety neurosis has a 50 per cent chance that his co-twin will be the same. Such evidence puts it beyond dispute that there is a genetic factor in abnormal anxiety. But this is not the whole answer, any more than it is with intelligence. Anxiety is not just inherited. There is too much evidence which points to the importance of early experience to draw this conclusion. Heredity and environment interact to produce their effects. However, as well as this, for abnormal anxiety to develop there must also be a set of precipitating circumstances.

Aggression

Unfortunately aggression seems to play an important part in human behaviour and it is of particular concern when it occurs in children. Consequently it will be the only other specific emotion to be discussed in detail in this chapter. Two of the important questions are whether or not people *need* to be aggressive from time to time and what is the effect of aggression and violence that they experience on the mass media?

Definitions

To begin with it is important to attempt to define aggression, since like all other aspects of emotion this is particularly difficult to do. If one person hits another the aggression involved is obvious, but sarcasm and other types of verbal aggression can be just as devastating as a physical blow. Also, over the years humans have devised all manner of subtle ways of expressing aggression indirectly, all of which have to be taken into account in a viable definition. For example, people are prone to gossip about one another, sometimes maliciously, they ignore one another, they are often inconsiderate, and so on.

The various types of human aggression can be analysed in Table 8.2.

Table 8.2: Types of Human Aggression

	Active		Passive	
	Direct	Indirect	Direct	Indirect
Physical	hitting	practical joke	sit-ins	refusing to do something
Verbal	insulting	malicious gossip	refusal to speak	refusing permission

The four types of aggression listed under 'passive' are clearly less extreme than those under 'active' but they are nevertheless aggressive acts.

Although this is a reasonably complete breakdown of aggression, there are still three important aspects which it leaves out. Each of these must be considered.

(1) Anger. Anger is certainly what a person feels when he is being aggressive. But aggression can occur without anger and anger can also lead to anxiety or depression as well as to aggression. Although any instance of aggression does involve delivering an unpleasant stimulus of some sort to another individual, people can hurt one another without anger being implicated. For example parents punish their children because they think it right to do so, without necessarily feeling angry

whilst so doing. And dentists drill their patients' teeth, presumably without anger although they might very well hurt them.

(2) Accident. People can deliver unpleasant or even harmful stimuli to one another accidentally. This is not aggression. If I trip up and send someone else flying, this is accident. Similarly, if I clumsily tip hot coffee over another person, this may be accident and is not an aggressive act.

(3) Intention. Unfortunately (for the psychologist) the only way to deal adequately with the difficulties made by anger and accident in defining aggression is to bring in the idea of intention. Aggression involves the intention to do harm, even if the act fails. If I aim a blow at someone and miss because of my own ineptitude it is still an aggressive act even though unsuccessful. But if I trip and in trying to save myself accidentally strike someone this is not aggression. In one case actual harm has been done (without aggression) and in the other no actual harm has been been caused (but the act is aggressive).

The problem comes with how to assess whether or not a person intends to be aggressive, or indeed intends to do anything. It is possible to ask a person his intentions but he might have good reasons for concealing them; he might not even know them if Freud's ideas on unconscious motivation are given credence. The only other possibility is to make close study of whatever led up to the aggressive act and whatever follows it. From this it is possible, although still difficult, to make inferences about intention.

Theories

The main theories of aggression apply equally well to childhood aggression as to adult aggression and have been concerned with how and why aggression occurs, and with what it does for people. There is supporting evidence of a sort for each of the theories, none of which as yet enables a decision to be made about which is the best.

Some theories of aggression stress *instinct* (blind, reflexive, unchanging behaviour), although as will be seen in the chapter on motivation it is very debatable whether man has instincts at all. Freud for example supposed that man has two basic instincts, a sexual, life-oriented force and an aggressive, death-oriented force. However much we try to control the aggressive instinct it keeps coming to the surface and causing overt aggression. Freud also suggested that aggression can be controlled by *catharsis* which literally means a purging. The idea is that if we have aggressive fantasies or see aggression in films or read of it in books, then this reduces our own inner aggression and makes it *less* likely that we will be openly aggressive. This idea (it is no more than an idea) has obvious relevance to the impact of televised aggression on children. The ethologist, Lorenz, holds similar ideas to those of Freud and argues that unless we have regular cathartic experiences, aggression will simply continue to well up within us until it overflows into what might look like aimless aggression.

A second theory suggests a relationship between *frustration* and aggression. The assumption is that aggression is an inbuilt reaction to frustration, to being thwarted in some way. If something persistently blocks you, you become angry and aggressive. If something you are trying to make simply will not come right, you smash it in anger, or if someone keeps being sarcastic to you and makes you seem to be something you are not you may eventually hit him. This theory would also be quite in line with the idea of aggression being dispelled cathartically.

Finally there is a theory of aggression based on *social learning*. This proposes that aggression is not innately determined or instinctual but is simply learned. Children learn to be aggressive by imitating aggression in adults and in other children, or by actually being aggressive and being rewarded for it. Such a viewpoint is clearly opposed to the idea of catharsis, proposing instead that aggression seen on the mass media or read about would simply lead to more aggression in an imitative manner. The idea is that there are *no* aggressive tendencies other than those which are learned or even taught.

As ever with theories of the origins of human behaviour there are the two camps represented; that which stresses genetic determinants and that which emphasises the environment and learning. Overall, particularly in studies of children there is no firm evidence to back up the instinctive theories of aggression. There is more evidence that aggression is learned by children. As far as televised aggression is concerned the evidence points both ways. Under some conditions, televised violence leads to more aggression in the observers, and in other conditions, to less. It remains an open question.

Anxiety and Aggression

One way in which psychologists have looked at the development of aggression is to put it together with anxiety. The argument runs as follows. If a child becomes aggressive to his parents then they might well be aggressive in return. He hits you and you hit him back, harder, and he stops. In fact, children tend to be punished aggressively more for aggression than for any other transgression. As seen before, one possible outcome of punishment is anxiety; a punished child is made anxious, thus associating one negative emotion with another: anxiety and anger. Thereafter, whenever the child feels angry and a resultant impulse to be aggressive, he will become anxious or worried.

As this is going on, the child is also developing techniques to deal with punishment. Punishment of aggression does not suppress it altogether, it simply makes it occur in more and more circumscribed situations. For this reason and many others, punishment is never the best technique for dealing with behaviour, particularly with aggressive behaviour. Especially as the child is being made to feel anxious rather than angry; there does not seem to be much to choose between the two as far as unpleasantness is concerned.

A final argument in this context is that extreme punishment will *not* inhibit aggression at all. It will induce frustration, one of the reactions to which is of course aggression. A child is aggressive; he is aggressively punished; he becomes frustrated and hence more aggressive; he is more aggressively punished: and so on until a complete breakdown in social relationships is the outcome.

Although these ideas are theoretical there is much in their favour, and a little supporting evidence. For example it has been shown that highly aggressive parents have highly aggressive children, but so do parents who are highly permissive towards their children's aggression. Non-aggressive children are to be found in families which steer a middle course between aggressive and permissive upbringing.

Conclusions

It should be clear by now that it is still impossible to give a simple definition of emotion; it is too complex a topic. It manifests itself at three distinct levels: bodily responses, overt behaviour, and subjective feelings and experiences. Each of these aspects has led to important theory and research with perhaps the best rapprochement between them being made by Izard (1972), although this is too complex to pursue here. Also, emotion seems to affect other non-emotional behaviour; it can lift it and increase its vigour or it can suppress and impede it. These effects occur in many different ways and situations which we learn to label in order to communicate about, and so we have the specific emotions.

Emotion provides the *quality* of our psychological functioning, colouring existence and making whatever is being done either seem worthwhile or pointless. Because it adds quality, emotion has been more difficult than other psychological capacities to quantify.

It is not possible to say which aspect of emotion is the most important; behaviour, physiological responses or cognition (with its attendant subjective feelings). Each would seem to be a necessary part of emotion, although at the everyday level it is probably its cognitive aspects which are the most important. However, for the psychologist these three levels of emotion lead to a two part problem. First, it is impossible for him to make a direct analysis of another person's subjective experience; at best, any information is only indirect and therefore open to bias. Secondly, what exactly is the role of subjective experience in emotion? Do they have a necessary, casual role to play, or do they simply go on in parallel to emotion's more overt aspects? Someone makes you angry, you lose your temper and strike him. Do your feelings of rage cause you to strike him? Does your striking of him cause your feeling of anger? Do the behaviour and the feelings simply go together as different faces of the same coin? These are important considerations since if the last of them is correct, then there is no need to study the subjective side of emotion, sufficient information can be gained by the study of its behavioural expression. At present all that can be said is that the cognitive and subjective aspects of emotion *seem* to be too important to be dropped from consideration.

Educating the Emotions

Although the present context is not appropriate for an extended discussion of psychotherapy, it is worth saying that in the last 15 or 20 years there has been an upsurge of interest in the psychological study of emotion and an increase in various types of therapy which have grown out of this. There seems to have been a growing concern for man's emotional problems. Emotions are less frequently seen as base primitive urges that interfere with purer reason. Now, emotion is seen more as an integral part of behaviour and experience.

This change in attitude has helped to lead the development of some interesting forms of therapy. For example, Izard (1972) describes the possiblity of treating emotional problems by training people in facial and bodily expressions which would inhibit the inappropriate ones which they tend to make socially. Arguably, however, this type of attitude should go much further; it might be important to educate both children and adults in emotional behaviour in just the way they are educated in other aspects of behaviour. Emotional education is something which typically has been ignored by society, and also by parents.

Usually, other than to train their children to cry less often, parents do very little about training the emotions. Educating people to work at their emotional lives as they work at other aspects of their lives could add an important dimension to their existence.

Summary Points

(1) Emotion is difficult to define, although it is clear that it involves behaviour, physiological responses, cognitions and subjective experience and that it occurs in particular (usually social) settings.

(2) Due to its complexity and to the problems of arousing it in artificial situations, emotion is notoriously difficult to study. However, many reasonably successful attempts have been made in research and theory which emphasise its different aspects.

(3) Early theories of emotion by James and Cannon have had a great influence, particularly in drawing attention to the importance of bodily processes in emotion and pointing to adaptive significance.

(4) Work on physiology and emotion has implicated various parts of the brain in emotion and has been very much concerned, although without much success, in the search for physiological response patterns which correspond to the various emotions.

(5) Very important contributions to an understanding of emotion have come from psychologists with a cognitive bias, particularly Schachter who shows the necessary roles in emotion taken by both physiology and cognition, the latter being important in the labelling of emotional states that we might experience. Also important in this context is the idea of appraisal – an instantaneous judgement that is made of the emotional significance of some event or stimulus.

(6) Work on emotional behaviour has been carried out very much within a framework of operant and classical conditioning and has involved some some rather complex methodology. Although very good from the scientific viewpoint, this work has not been especially productive of good theory, and some people would argue that it is rather a long way removed from emotion as we know it.

(7) Anxiety exemplifies the study of abnormal emotion and has probably been more studied than any other single emotion. Typical theories distinguish between neurotic and objective anxiety and between anxiety as a temporary state and anxiety as a more long-lasting trait. Work on the causes of anxiety are caught between the same heredity-environment problem as is often seen in developmental psychology. It is still not possible to say whether anxiety is a genuine state of the

organism with casual roles in behaviour or merely a description of some rather complex behavioural and bodily response.

(8) Various problems remain for the psychologist in the study of emotion, particularly with respect to what status he should assign to cognitions and subjective experiences. However, an argument can be made made that increasing interest in emotion should promote society to pay more attention to its use in educational contexts.

Study Question – 8

(1) What examples of aggression and anger have you seen amongst your patients? Are you sure that they were instances of aggression rather than accidents? Or rather than of some other condition?

(2) When thinking about the emotional lives of your patients and your colleagues do you find greater understanding from the behavioural, the physiological or the cognitive sides of it? Which do you think to be the most important aspect of emotion?

(3) What are the predominant emotions of everyday life? What are the situations which most commonly bring them about?

(4) Do you think that illness and hospitalisation carry with them particular emotional problems? What are they? Why do they come about?

(5) From your observations of yourself and of others, it is likely that you have recognised the importance of the subjective experience of emotion. How is it possible to determine what emotion another person (particularly a patient) is experiencing?

(6) How important a role has been played by anxiety in your own life and studies? How important is the anxiety which is often expressed by people who are in hospitals, and what could be done to alleviate it?

(7) How much attention do you think that you should pay to the emotional reactions of your patients?

(8) As part of your professional work in a hospital, do you think that you would ever need to educate your patients emotionally? How would you go about this?

(9) To what extent do you think that all the problems of abnormal behaviour or mental disorder are really emotional in origin?

(10) Write a thorough profile of the emotional life of a patient or a colleague whom you know particularly well. Attempt to show how any changes in the person's emotional reactions are related to his experiences, his successes and his failures.

9 MOTIVATION

Impetus for Behaviour

Activity is an inevitable corollary of life. All organisms are active, this activity reaching its greatest variability and flexibility at the human level. But activity is not aimless; it is rarely one can observe an animal moving around in its environment without also seeing that it is moving *towards* or *away from* something. Often it appears to be seeking some goal. Goal-seeking is the most basic aspect of behaviour which motivation has been used to *explain*, although as will become clear later it is difficult to determine the extent to which motivation merely provides a *description* of behaviour.

As well as to account for goal-directed behaviour, psychologists have also emphasised the concept of motivation for other reasons. Consider for example the state which most persons experience from time to time, that of not having spoken to another human being for hours or even days. They deal with such social deprivation in a multitude of ways, each of which leads to the goal of social contact. The idea of social motivation helps to gather together and to account for this variety of means of achieving a single end. A further point is that some stimuli seem to impel us to immediate action, rather in the way that a trigger sets off the firing mechanism of a gun. Think, for example, of a knock at the door or of the shrill of the telephone. What gives such stimuli their special significance? In what ways do they differ from other stimuli? The idea of motivation helps to answer such questions.

Definitions

Before discussing motivation any further, it would perhaps be useful to define the terms which are most commonly used by those who work in this area.
(1) *Needs* are deficiencies in something that the organism requires for survival; food or oxygen, for example.
(2) *Drives* refer either to the energising motives which are related to biological needs (physiological drives) or to the secondary or derived motives (psychological drives) which are believed to develop through learning on the basis of association with physiological drives.
(3) *Motives* are conditions of the organism which give it energy channelled in particular directions, i.e. towards particular goals.

152

(4) *Motivation* is a broader term than those above, a concept which links needs, drive and motives and which is also used to refer to the general energised state of an organism.

(These are approximate definitions. In practice, the terms need, drive, and motive are often applied interchangeably, particularly in general writing about psychology.)

Problems

There are a number of problems which any analysis of the role of motivation in behaviour must consider. The first and perhaps the most important concerns the idea that some motives are *basic* to humanity. If this is so, then it would seem reasonable to attempt to ascribe motives to the behaviour of other people. Throughout the history of thought in philosophy and psychology the notion that some motives are basic to man has been expressed in a number of ways. For example, the Greeks and Romans saw man as a pawn of the gods, being given his motivation by them; then, during the Renaissance, man was viewed as a freely choosing master of his own fate. Darwin's influence turned the tables a little by laying emphasis on the similarity between the motives of man and the animals, and then Freud added another, and rather confusing, dimension by drawing attention to the importance of unconscious motives in determining what people do.

Each of these views has some merit and, surprisingly enough, each is still held in some quarters of society. The existence of such a variety of viewpoints means that extreme care has to be taken in ascribing motives to other people. One should be reticent in saying – 'he did that because . . . ', particularly in view of the doubt about whether one was attempting to explain his behaviour or merely to describe it.

One of the better descriptions of the way in which motivation in real life is conceptualised at present is given by McGregor (1960). He suggests that everyday human motivation is seen in two ways.
(1) Traditional – humans do not like work; they must be threatened into doing it; they like being directed; they dislike responsibility.
(2) Integrative – it is natural to make effort, as it is to rest; humans can control themselves; they become committed to objectives if rewarded for it; they can accept responsibility; many persons are creative and ingenious; industrial life is not especially fulfilling intellectually. Which of these two broad views is nearer to the truth is impossible to say.

A second problem is that, like memories, motives are constructs used both by psychologists and the layman. All that we can ever observe directly is behaviour, and we sometimes use our observation to make inferences about motives. For example, if we see an infant to be crying and irritable and observe that it has not been fed for some hours, then we assume it to be hungry and feed it. But, however well-founded these assumptions seem to be, it is still only an assumption. Hunger cannot be *observed*, it can only be inferred from other things; it may be that the baby is crying because a pin is sticking into it.

So, the observation and measurement of motivation is a problem. We *can* see behaviour apparently directed towards some goals rather than others, to food rather than water for instance. And we *can* observe signs of satiation, a normal animal will stop eating after a time and direct its attention elsewhere. However, even these observations are difficult to make with the more obviously psychological rather than physiological motives. Just to give one example for the moment, think of the plenitude of ways in which it is possible to be ambitious; prediction is virtually impossible.

Measurement

Bearing in mind the difficulties just mentioned, psychologists have devised four main ways of measuring drives, particularly in animals.
(1) *General activity* : the speed at which an animal runs in an activity cage or wheel, for example, can be related to hours for which it has been deprived of some necessity of life such as food.
(2) *Rate* of performing a learned act. This is more rapid when hungry (up to a point) and less rapid when sated.
(3) *Overcoming obstructions* : for example, the degree of shock a food-deprived rat will take in crossing an electrified floor to get to food provides a measure of the strength of his hunger drive.
(4) *Choice* : given a choice between, say, food and water, the direction of choice is assumed to indicate which of the drives is the stronger.

Notice that each of these methods of measuring drive is indirect. It is worth re-emphasising the point that it is impossible to observe motivation directly or to look at a drive directly.

Instincts

A final general problem of motivation concerns instinct, a term which was once very widely used amongst psychologists. Nowadays, psychologists rarely use it, although in the everyday world it is bandied about freely. Instincts were defined (somewhat similarly to motives) as being propensities of the organism to perceive the world selectively and to pursue a biologically useful line of behaviour. But these propensities were thought to be innate, complex and common to all the members of a species.

In spite of McDougall's (1908) powerful arguments to the contrary, there is *no* good evidence for their existence in humans, although there is some indication that they exist in animals. However, even at the animal level instinct is a dangerous concept, hinting strongly as it does at explanation without really providing any. It is of no help to say that a spider builds a web because it has an instinct to build a web. This is merely circular, and the circle cannot be broken without saying what the instinct is, how it comes about, how it can be influenced, and so on; in other words, without saying what *really* makes the spider build its web.

Characteristics of Motivated Behaviour

Finally, by way of a general introduction, motivated behaviour, and therefore perhaps *all* behaviour, has four main characteristics.
(1) It is *instigated*, from some deficit within the organism or from some external incentive. Hunger, for example, might be aroused from pangs in the gut and/or from the sight and smell of food.
(2) It is *directional*, the instigated behaviour goes towards or away from something for obvious reasons, a movement towards being easier to recognise than a movement away.
(3) It is *selective*. A food-deprived animal seems to be dominated by its hunger; everything is perceived and interpreted in that way.
(4) It is *satiable*. When a goal is attained, the behaviour changes and the organism becomes less restless. This is easy to see with the basic needs. Think for example of what you do after a large meal; it needs no description. Satiation is less clear with social motives. For example, is an ambitious or power-hungry person ever satisfied? There is some indication that the more complex social motives develop their own autonomy and therefore continue after any initial goals have been reached.

Needs: Physiological Drives and Motives

(1) Hunger

The hunger drive has a well-defined physiological basis, although as will become clear there is more to hunger than cues which come solely from the body. The obvious cue to hunger comes from contractions of a relatively empty stomach, such contractions being related to the 'pangs' of hunger which we all experience. This relationship was shown in a number of early studies which involved subjects swallowing balloons which were then inflated against the stomach walls. A tube from the balloon led out through the mouth and was connected to a recording instrument so that a record could be made of contractions. These contractions were found to coincide reasonably well with subjective reports of hunger pangs.

However, the physiology of hunger is more complex than this. If the sensory nerves (of rats) which run from the stomach to the brain are cut, the animals continue to seek for food in much the same way as usual. It may therefore be that the brain interprets changes in the blood stream as well as taking account of stomach contractions. This idea is supported by work implicating the *hypothalamus* in hunger. If the ventromedial nucleus of the hypothalamus is removed (normally by being burnt out with a special electrode) an animal will literally eat itself to death, becoming enormously fat, a condition known as hyperphagia. Alternatively, if the lateral nucleus is removed the animal will starve to death; aphagia. These nuclei would appear to be centres which control eating and food satiation.

Everyday observation shows that people differ in their food preferences, that is, they develop what are called *specific hungers*. Davis, 1928, for example, gave young children a free choice of a very wide range of foods. He found that if they were allowed this freedom of choice, and if the experimenters tolerated any sort of mess, then over a period of time the children chose a balanced diet. Of course, in the short term it did not appear to be well balanced. If young infants can regulate their needs in this way, there must be specific physiological mechanisms involved, although these have not yet been found. The problem is complicated further in that if older people are given this free choice of what to eat, then they sometimes choose a very unbalanced diet. Presumably, they have learned to have preferences which in excess are not good for them.

As well as being aroused by physiological cues, hunger is also dependent on cues *outside* the organism, as recent work by Schachter (e.g. 1971) has demonstrated. In a series of real-life and laboratory studies on obesity, Schachter showed that in comparison with persons of normal weight, the obese eat far more in response to external stimuli such as the sight and smell of food and the time of day it happens to be. Although persons of normal weight are also responsive to such stimuli, they are more dependent than the obese on physiological cues.

As an example of the research on which these ideas are based, Schachter and Gross (1968) found that obese persons who have been deceived about the passage of time eat more than similarly deceived persons of normal weight when they believe it to be later than it actual actually is, and less when they believe it to be earlier. Similarly, Goldman, Jaffa and Schachter (1968) found that obese Jews are more likely to fast on Yom Kippur than are Jews of normal weight. In each case the implication is that the obese person is more dependent on external influences.

The *selective and directional* effects of hunger are well established and easily exemplified by Sandford (1936). He deprived subjects of food for a few hours and then showed them a series of ambiguous blobs and shapes. In comparison with subjects not deprived of food, the experimental subjects saw many more food and food-related objects in the ambiguous material.

Also, it is well established that persons who, from their own choice or through environmental rigours, stay for long periods on semi-starvation diets, become very single-mindedly oriented to food. Even their reading becomes centred on cookery books, recipes and diet sheets. It is as if their hunger drive has taken over their intellectual lives.

In the extreme a continuing state of semi-starvation can result in apparent changes in personality, even though these might be only temporary. For example, the person's sex-drive wanes, if not disappearing altogether, and he becomes irritable, apathetic, humourless, and depressed. Everything seems to give way to the predominant state of hunger.

Finally, there is the question of what makes an organism stop eating once it has started. There must be some mechanism which controls this, otherwise, like the hyperphagic rats, once we start eating, we would go on for ever. It was pointed out earlier that satiation has some basis in chemical changes within the body, particularly the hypothalamus, but once again, the matter is more complex than this. Animals and humans often eat when, from the bodily point of view, there is absolutely no *need* to, and naturally, as a result they become overweight. Eating then is definitely of psychological as well as physiological significance. Food means more than just bodily nourishment, and it is work such as Schachter's which is beginning to provide information about this psychological significance.

(2) Thirst

The history of research into the thirst drive is very similar to that of hunger, so it will be dealt with more briefly, the relevant early work being well reviewed by Cofer and Appley (1964). At the simplest level, thirst would appear to depend on the salivary glands becoming insufficiently moist for comfort, the resulting dryness leading the organism to seek water. But again, this simple level does not provide explanation enough. For example, many animals (e.g. birds) do not have salivary glands, and dogs with the appropriate sensory nerves cut continue to drink.

Another possibility is that thirst results from an overall deficit in the amount of water in the body, only one reflection of which is in the salivary glands. This idea is supported by work on dogs which have had their mouths bypassed with gastric fistulas. The dogs are then deprived of water for some hours and water is finally put directly into their stomachs. If time is allowed for the body to absorb this, the dogs do not drink if given the opportunity.

This way of looking at the thirst drive is also not enough to account for all the facts. Thus the current viewpoint is that thirst results from a deficit in the amount of water in the body in relation to the amount of salt. As with the hunger drive, it has been established that certain areas of the hypothalamus are implicated in the control of thirst, but at present the exact processes are unknown.

The more psychological aspects of thirst parallel those of hunger. A water-deprived person will be dominated by thirst to the exclusion of all else; the portrayal of this in films of desert treks is based on fact. Similarly, there is some evidence that a physiological/neurological mechanism acts to control the cessation of drinking. But, as with hunger, there are many instances of both people and animals drinking far more than bodily balance dictates. Certainly, the amount of water which passes through the mouth and enters the stomach is relevant to satiation, but if the water is sweetened for example then many species will take far more than they would otherwise. And of course the adulteration of water with alchohol has similar effects on its intake in humans.

(3) Sex

The third drive which has a basis in physiological need is sex, which differs from hunger and thirst in that it is germane to species survival rather than to the survival of the individual. Also, although it does depend on physiological processes, its influence by learning is much more apparent than it is in hunger and thirst, particularly in humans.

In the human male the pituitary gland is crucial to the physiology of sex. And obviously the testes are implicated through their dual function of secreting androgens (male sex hormones) into the blood stream, and of producing sperm. The strength of the sex drive depends *partly* on androgen quality and reaches a peak in the late teens. On average, and given the opportunity, the frequency of sexual behaviour is three times per week at ages 16-25, two and a half times at 30, twice at 40 and once at 60. However, if the androgens are not produced (after castration, for example) but sexual behaviour has already been learned, it does not cease or alter. This implies that in some (unknown) sense the brain takes over from the testes.

A similar pattern to this is also seen in the physiological arousal of the human female sex drive. The pituitary gland is involved and the ovaries secrete oestrogen which influences the sexual urge. In the female, sexual receptivity and desire is at its nadir during ovulation and reaches its zenith immediately before and after menstruation. A general point which is worth making about human sexuality is that no frequency is normal. This comes from a survey by Hunt (1974) in which he found sexual behaviour to occur more than once per day in some cases to less than once per year in others. Also, the question of selectivity is very similar to that seen for hunger and thirst, the sexually aroused person is little interested in food, drink, or indeed anything other than the gratification of sexual needs.

Knowledge concerning the satiation of the sex drive is very confused. In males it is clear that the major goal of sex is ejaculation. This is always followed by a refractory period when interest and ability (in sex) have declined, often to nothing; then there is a gradual increase in proclivity. However, there are large individual differences in the length of the refractory period, which also depends on social (learned) factors, such as the presence of a new and stimulating partner, for example.

In their major survey of the human sexual response. Masters and Johnson (1966) produced some interesting facts about sexual satiation in females. For example, up to 25 per cent of women do not experience orgasms although apparently still enjoying sex, and even though all women are capable of it. Some women have a number of orgasms in rapid succession, such capacities being limited by the capabilities of their partners. Also, it was found that there is only one type of female orgasm, not the clitoral and vaginal as was once supposed.

Again it is Masters and Johnson (1970) who point to the efficacy of sexual therapy for persons who have sexual problems. Such therapy has been carried out successfully on many thousands of people and has led to the unequivocal rejection of several sexual myths. For example:
(a) The intact hymen is no proof of virginity; and its absence is not proof of non-virginity;
(b) There is no good medical reason for avoiding sexual intercourse

during menstruation;
(c) Sterilisation neither enhances nor impedes sexual behaviour and enjoyment;
(d) There is no need to avoid sex during pregnancy;
(e) There is generally no optimum position for sexual enjoyment;
(f) Oral-genital sex does not indicate latent homosexuality.
(Examples taken from Kaats and Davis, 1972.)

(4) Pain

Yet again, pain brings about a drive which has both physiological and psychological components. At the crudest level, pain is the result of tissue damage or stress which induces a need to reduce the intense stimulation it brings about. Not only is this stimulation subjectively unpleasant but it is also a warning of danger to the organism. The escape from, and avoidance of, pain takes very many forms, ranging from a simple reflex to complex behaviour such as attending a hospital or taking medication.

When bodily tissue is damaged or stressed this instigates nervous impulses to the spinal cord and then back to the muscles and/or up to the brain. But pain is not merely a neurological matter; reactions to it are often modified by learning. For example, a sportsman who injures himself whilst playing his sport may well not notice the injury or feel any pain until after the match. Also, think of the many ways of dealing with pain, from putting on a bandage to walking carefully to favour an injury — all such reactions must be learned. And finally, there seem to be cultural or sub-cultural differences in the tolerance of pain. In western society for example there are male/female differences, these presumably being learned early in life.

(5) Exploration

The final drive which is usually included within the physiological bracket is exploration. The reason for this inclusion is that exploratory behaviour and curiosity appear to be unlearned in many species. However, as yet nothing is known about any physiological deficits which lead to it; the physiology of exploration remains uncharted.

There are of course psychological influences on exploratory behaviour. For example, animals explore more in complex than in simple environments, they explore more when young than when old, more when unafraid than when afraid, and, given a choice, they tend to *choose* complex rather than simple environments. That most of the higher animals explore is obvious, but in the absence of an observable physiological basis for this, whether or not it is appropriate to include it within a group of physiological needs is moot.

Psychological Motives

Psychological motives are far more complex than the more primary physiological needs. This is perhaps because they are almost entirely learned, probably as a development from physiological needs, and the possibilities of learning in humans are virtually endless. For the most part, psychological motives are concerned with the intricacies of personality and social behaviour.

The complexities bring an extra series of difficulties to the study of human motivation, not least of which are those concerned with whether or not such motivation actually exists, and if so how to measure it. For instance there is no firm evidence that young children have any motive to be dominant, but it is obvious that many adults behave dominantly. Is motivation involved? If so, how does it come about?

Also, psychological motives are difficult to choose. For example, if during a social interaction person A is sarcastic to person B, is this because A has a grouse against the world, a grouse against B, has been hurt by B, has a career or a home life that is going wrong, has a tooth-ache, or what? Yet a classification of typology of psychological drives has to be attempted if the idea of psychological motivation is to have theoretical value. From the view point of explanation, it would be useless to invoke a new motive to account for every bit of behaviour that was observed, for then, to say that a person did something because he was motivated so to do would be to say no more than he did it.

One motive that does seem to be psychologically distinct from others and which has consequently received much attention is the so-called *need* (this should really be drive) *to achieve*, usually referred to as nAch. Some of the work on nAch will be discussed as an example of the general approach to psychological motivation. It has been developed by Atkinson (e.g. 1958), Heckhausen (e.g. 1967) and particularly McClelland (e.g. 1961).

nAch can be defined as 'a condition which energises the organism to seek for itself high levels of performance in various situations'. Notice that this definition draws attention to the *seeking* of achievements, the implication being that a person with high nAch will not *necessarily* be one *who has* achieved a great deal. The thematic apperception test (TAT) allows a form of quantitative assessment of nAch. This involves subjects telling stories about four pictures (representing man and machine, boy at desk, father and son, and boy day-dreaming.) The stories are then scored by independent judges as to the number of achievement-related themes they contain. This method is believed to reveal the degree to which a person strives for excellence, a condition of which he himself may not be fully aware. However, TAT judgements are not of good reliability and they can only be used to make group rather than individual assessments.

Research has shown nAch to be related to type of upbringing, high nAch being seen especially in those persons who are trained to be independent at a relatively early age; that is, those who could for example entertain themselves and deal with their own pocket money and clothes earlier than the average. On the other hand, adults who have low nAch scores tend to have had mothers who expected independence much later. However, high nAch does not develop in children who become independent through being left alone; apparently the independence has to be encouraged and rewarded with physical affection. There is also tentative evidence that similar relationships between nAch and upbringing exist in a number of different societies.

Research has also been carried out into the selectivity of nAch, tending to support the idea that it does give the high scorer a definite direction in what he does. For example, tachistoscopic studies have shown that high nAch scorers are particularly sensitive to (have lowered thresholds to) achievement words. Also, with IQ matched, high nAch scorers outperform low scorers on many tasks; they are constantly oriented to do well. nAch is also related to the taking of moderate, calculated risks rather than to the showing of great daring.

This brief discussion has only skimmed the surface of the considerable amount of work on achievement motivation. Many of its facets have been studied. Comparisions have been made between males and females, for example. In western cultures for instance females are often (although not always of course) characterised by a fear of success and a will to fail, perhaps because they have been brought up to believe that success may lead them to lose friends and to be less attractive otherwise. Most extremely, achievement motivation has been speculatively related to economic advances and recessions in different societies at various periods in their evolution. Such historical research can of course only be speculative (see McClelland, 1961).

Naturally, psychological motives other than achievement have been studied, those concerned with power, dominance and affiliation for example. Research in these areas has not been especially noteworthy, however. The exception to this can perhaps be found in studies of human aggression, a discussion of which can be found in chapter 8.

Classification of Motives

The remaining aspect of motivation which has received serious psychological study concerns the possibility of classifying motives, especially at the human level. If you remember, this exercise is important if motives are not to lose their meaning and explanatory usefulness by being overproliferated.

Arguably, the most interesting and best conceived classification of motives came from Maslow's (e.g. 1954, 1972) hierarchy. His basic system contains five types of motivation:

(a) *physiological* needs of the sort described earlier,

(b) motives based on *safety*, the drive to feel secure, to have somewhere to live and to minimise risks in life,

(c) the drive to *belong* to others, to feel loved or liked by them,

(d) the drive for *esteem,* to have the respect and admiration of others,

(e) the drive to *self-actualisation*, to gain optimal self-fulfilment and self-realisation from life, to be content with and to gain maximum satisfaction from one's life and interests.

Later, Maslow added two further types of motivation between d) and e). These were drives to achieve *cognitive* satisfaction and to be gratified *aesthetically.*

The important point about Maslow's classification is that he conceived it as a hierarchy. This means that if motives at any one level are not satisfied then the person is stuck at that level, he cannot move up the hierarchy. So, for example, if a man is concerned with providing himself and his family with somewhere to live, he will be unconcerned with a feeling of belonging and unworried by the esteem of others. Or if a person is wrapped up in deriving esteem from others he cannot become self-actualised. In general, Maslow argued that motives lower in the hierarchy are more potent than the higher ones; there can be no concern with the higher motives if the lower motives remain unsatisfied.

Although Maslow's hierarchy of motives is convincingly described, the evidence to support it is less convincing. This evidence is positive enough at the first two levels (physiology and safety) even amongst animals, but moving up the hierarchy, the evidence amounts to little more than Maslow's observations of life. Even though these observations were made systematically, they are still open to the many biases to which any everyday observation must be subject.

A final question posed by considering the classification of motives is whether or not there exist some motives which can be relied upon, that will be observed in human action time and time again. For this to be so a motive would have to have a discernible physiological or chemical basis, to be seen throughout the animal kingdom up to and including the human species in which it would have to occur in all the members. Clearly, physiological needs would meet these criteria, but it is of the more psychological motives that the question is asked. Of these, the only one which comes near is aggression. Were aggression to be proved to have this dependable universality, it would be a depressing thought. However, evidence for its ubiquitousness comes mainly from Lorenz's (1966) argument and very biased selection of samples. At best, the dependability of the aggression motive is debatable (see Chapter 8).

Summary Points

(1) Motivation is a psychological construct. It cannot be observed directly and must be inferred from behaviour.
(2) The physiological needs are hunger, thirst, sex, pain and exploration. In one way or another they are basic to individual and/or species survival and have both physiological (built-in) and psychological (learned) components.
(3) It is difficult to be sure whether or not psychological motives exist. On the assumption that they do, most work has been done on achievement motivation which seems to be linked to upbringing and family experience.
(4) Some attempts have been made to classify motives, the most notable of which is Maslow's, which places human motives in a clearly defined hierarchical order.

Study Questions – 9

(1) Do you find it easy to interpret the needs, wishes, desires, and general motivations of your patients? What do you think causes these motivations?
(2) Do you think that either the general or the specific motivations of people who are in hospital or have been injured are systematically different from those of other people? What are the main motives of hospital patients?
(3) How would you measure the strength of a patient's hunger? How would you assess how much pain he is feeling?
(4) How would you attempt to motivate someone to overcome an injury, an illness, or some other handicap?
(5) How would you deal with a patient who seeks too much attention?

How would you stop him irritating other patients by doing so?

(6) From what you have seen in your training and in your professional experiences, do you think that some motives, such as 'competitiveness' are 'human nature'? What does this phrase mean?

(7) What do you think makes some people lose their motivation in life? Does this happen more or less in a hospital setting than in the outside world?

(8) How would you motivate a young child to take a course of action which he found to be unpleasant but which you knew to be necessary to his health and development?

(9) Compare any two patients known to you, one highly successful in overcoming his difficulties, the other unsuccessful. What are the motivational differences between them? Do the same for any two of your colleagues.

(10) Do you think that Maslow's hierarchy of motives can apply to your patients as well as it might to other people? Is it possible for someone with an illness or disability to be self-actualised? If so, are all such a person's 'lower' motives satisfied before this occurs?

10 PERSONALITY THEORY

There have been very many definitions of personality, ranging from: 'Personality is behaviour' to 'Personality is the sum total of all the biological innate dispositions, impulses, tendencies, appetites and instincts of the individual, and the acquired dispositions and tendencies'. Neither of these definitions is particularly helpful. Perhaps the best working definition is that of Allport (1961) who states that personality is the . . . 'unique organisation of enduring attributes of the individual'.

This definition points clearly to what the study of personality is about, be it theoretical or empirical. It involves the study of the *whole* person over some time, and not just the sort of brief sample of some small aspect of his behaviour as would be studied in the laboratory. When this is done, three points become apparent. (1) Behaviour tends to be *consistent* from one situation to the next and people are reasonably predictable as to their aggression, or dominance, or anxiety, etc. (2) A person's behaviour seems to be *organised*. He seems to function as a system with his own style and individual patterns of behaviour. (3) Some aspects of a person's behaviour are *unique*.

As with so many concepts in psychology, personality is intangible. It cannot be pointed to or touched, but can only be determined by influence. Also, its measurement can only be indirect. Personality is an abstraction, not a directly observed phenomenon. It is a hypothetical construct which intervenes somewhere between stimulus and response, between the environment and behaviour, and which some psychologists believe to affect behaviour.

It should be clear from this brief description that the psychologist views personality quite differently from the layman. Certainly the layman stresses the uniqueness of the individual but he also tends to speak of personality as an *overall* characteristic or quality that some people have more or less of than others. He will talk of much or of little personality and will emphasise consistency.

Psychologists, although definitely not defining personality in this way, do in fact study it from many different viewpoints and with various emphases; and they develop numerous theories as a result. Each personality theorist tends to use different constructs and to emphasise different facets of what is a complex subject. Each of these might be (partially) correct. The remainder of this chapter will be spent in describing some of the major theories of personality, chosen because they exemplify the various viewpoints and because they have been fairly influential. The main vantage points will be: constitutional, developmental, the self and experience, behavioural, and psychometric.

Constitution: Sheldon (1942, 1954)

The best known constitutional theory of personality was put forward by Sheldon, whose basic belief was that people can be classified into a limited number of personality *types* and that these types relate to a similar classification of body types. He argued that it is possible to take measures of a person's *basic* body type; genetically determined and unaffected by environmental influences such as illness or dieting. He felt that personality type develops as a *result* of body type.

Typically, Sheldon rated people on three seven-point scales with respect to their major bodily characteristics. He labelled the extremes on these dimensions as:

endomorphy	— fat, soft, non-muscular.
mesomorphy	— stocky, broad, muscular.
ectomorphy	— thin, bony, fragile.

He assessed personality similarly on three seven point scales. The extremes of the personality dimensions were labelled:

viscerotonia	— happy-go-lucky, jolly, equable, generous etc.
somatotonia	— aggressive, tough-minded, competitive, etc.
cerebrotonia	— thoughtful, aesthetic, intellectual, etc.

Of course, even with this typology, Sheldon is not saying that everyone in the world is divisible into three body and personality classes. People vary in *degree* of the *three* body types and personality types. But he is saying that body type leads to or causes personality type. Also, although his means of gathering evidence have been shown to be questionable, he did describe some striking correlations between physique and personality.

However, even if it is established that physique and personality are related there are other possible reasons for this than the causal link which Sheldon suggests. (1) Bias may have influenced Sheldon's results, since the one set of observers rated both body type and personality type and they were aware of Sheldon's hypotheses. (2) Many people hold stereotypes about the relationship between physique and personality. This could well have the effect of pushing people with particular builds into behaving in particular ways, according to the stereotype. (3) It could be that whatever complex factors cause personality to develop, also lead to the development of particular body types.

Overall, even if there is some relationship between physique and personality, a typology of personality which classifies people into a limited number of types tends to be forcing the issue rather too much. It could be pushing something which is naturally complex into an artificial oversimplification.

Development: 1 Freud

It is important to spend some time describing Freud's (e.g. 1946) theory of personality since it has probably been more influential than any other. It was the first psychoanalytic theory and also highlights the effects of biological and family influences. In-built motives determine the extent and direction of behaviour, and this lays the groundwork for the developing personality.

Freud suggested that the personality is made up of three mental systems, each with its own energy.

(1) The id. This is the basic, biological system with which we are born and which provides energy for the other systems. The principle which underlies it is tension reduction which is achieved by *reflex actions* (e.g. eye blinks) which bring immediate relief, and the *primary process* which reduces tension through a wish-fulfilling generation of images of a desired object. Discharge of tension in the id produces pleasure.

(2) The ego. The ego allows us to live in the objective world. Its basic means of action is the *reality principle* which prevents the discharge of energy until an appropriate object is found. Fundamentally, the ego has executive functions, both selecting aspects of the environment to which we should respond and integrating the other two energy systems. It mediates between the external environment and the id, and receives its energy from the id.

(3) The superego. This system is concerned with the internalisation of cultural and moral standards. Wrong acts are punished thereby leading to the development of the *conscience* and right acts are approved thereby leading to the development of the *ego-ideal.* Via these mechanisms, the superego suppresses socially unacceptable urges of the id, diverts the ego from realistic goals to those which are morally approved, and strives

to perfection. The superego is fighting both the id and the ego.

Freud's emphasis on the importance of development to personality also points to a three part process which centres on the mouth, the anus and the genitalia, the three erogenous zones of the body. His general argument is that the basic needs associated with these areas are important for the developing personality. Each is a source of irritation and excitation which has to be dealt with. Each also leads to conflicts with parents and therefore to frustrations and anxieties.

(1) Oral zone. In the infant, according to Freud, erotic and aggressive pleasure come from tactual stimulation and biting. The mouth has five functions each of which provides a prototype for a personality trait;
(a) taking in — acquisitiveness,
(b) holding on — tenacity,
(c) biting — destructiveness,
(d) spitting out — rejection/contempt,
(e) closing — refusal and negation.
The precise personality development depends on whatever frustrations and anxieties are associated with the prototype, fixation on any one possibly leading to a complete range of interests, attitudes and values.

(2) Anal zone. Here there is tension from accumulated faecal material, expulsion of which brings relief. Also, toilet training in the second year or thereabouts almost always has some emotional aspects to it. Freud saw this as involving a conflict between instinct (get rid of it anywhere at any time) and external control (get rid of it here and now). For example a child trained harshly may purposely soil himself and as an adult become messy, irresponsible, disorderly, wasteful or extravagant. Or the child may react against the harsh training and become an adult who is meticulous, disgusted, or frugal.

If toilet training is achieved through pleading and praising, the child may develop into a generous, philanthropic adult. Or, if this type of training makes the child feel that he has lost something valuable, he may become a depressed, depleted, anxious adult. Or he may refuse to give up his valuable faeces and become a thrifty, parsimonious, economical adult. All of which is very interesting but covers so many possibilities that it cannot be used as a basis for prediction.

(3) Sexual zone. The next stage in Freud's theory of personality development revolves around the genital region. In boys this takes the form of the *oedipus complex*. Briefly, a boy loves his mother and

identifies with his father. As his sexual urges increase between the ages of three and five, he develops an incestuous love for his mother and jealousy of his father. Also he may suffer from castration anxiety in which he feels that his father might remove his penis. This is brought home to him if and when he sees the sexual anatomy of a girl. He then represses his incestuous desire for his mother and hatred of his father. The oedipus complex disappears due to this repression, maturation, and its overall impossibility.

The female sexual stage is dominated by the *electra complex.* Early on in life a girl loves her mother but does not identify with her father. She begins to blame her mother for her lack of male sex organs, and generally comes to prefer her father, although this is mixed with envy of him (penis envy). She comes to love her father and be jealous of her mother. The electra complex according to Freud becomes weaker with time, but never completely disappears.

For both sexes, from the age of about five until puberty, sexual problems are not apparent; this is the *latency* period.

This brief description is only sufficient to give an idea of Freud's very complex personality theory. Its strength is that, apart from descriptions of personality, particularly the abnormal, it is concerned with 'why' and 'how' questions and searches for dynamics which might underlie personality. Although widely discussed and very influential, many criticisms can be levelled against it. For example:

(1) The three systems of personality cannot easily be observed or measured; they are sheerly hypothetical mental apparatus. Ultimately, it is a question of either believing in their existence or not, rather than being able to prove the point one way or the other.

(2) Freud's descriptions and explanations come from pathological rather than normal individuals, and even the pathological patients he studied were few in number. Can the theory therefore be applied to the normal personality? It is difficult to say.

(3) Freud overemphasised unconscious processes without any justification for so doing.

(4) Perhaps the worst aspect of Freud's theory is that it has led to attempts to incorporate psychoanalysis into a scientific framework. This is nonsensical since psychoanalysis is essentially unquantifiable. However, to end on a more positive note, Freud's theory was significant in its reliance on principles of cause and effect and its emphasis on personality being the product of an individual's history.

Development: 2 Erikson (1963)

Erikson is usually described as a neo-Freudian and has a theory of personality even more obviously developmental than Freud's. He certainly pays attention to a greater span of development than Freud, arguing for example, that an adolescent has to develop an identity, control sexual urges and establish a proper self; all of which influences personality. Erikson builds his stages of personality development around the ego, which is adaptive oriented to reality, and based on energy for learning.

Erikson describes eight significant stages in the development of personality, each of which involves important conflicts, and each of which leads to the development of particular aspects of personality.
(1) A sense of trust versus mistrust. This achieves *hope* and occurs in the equivalent of Freud's oral stage.
(2) A sense of autonomy versus doubt and shame. This leads to the development of *will*, occurring in Freud's anal stage.
(3) A sense of initiative versus guilt, leading to the development of *purpose* and occurring in the genital stage.
(4) A sense of industry versus inferiority, leading to the development of *competence* and occurring in the latency period.
(5) A sense of identity versus identity diffusion, leading to the development of fidelity and occurring in puberty and adolescence.
(6) A sense of intimacy and solidarity versus isolation, leading to the development of *love* and occurring in young adulthood.
(7) A sense of generativity versus self-absorption and stagnation, leading to the development of *care*, in adulthood.
(8) A sense of integrity versus despair or disgust, leading to the development of *wisdom* and occurring at maturity.

As with Freud, Erikson would argue that if anything goes wrong at any of these conflict stages there would be problems for the developing personality. Also, many of the same criticisms which are levelled at Freud can also be levelled at Erikson, and indeed at any of the neo-Freudians.

The Self: 1 Rogers

There are a number of personality theories which centre around ideas such as the self. They reject the dynamic and motivational concepts of psychoanalytical theory and the assumptions of many other types of theory. They illustrate the phenomenological and existential theories in emphasising immediate experience and perceptions. The individual is seen as an experiencing being who has important subjective experiences which must be explored if he is to be understood.

Rogers' (e.g. 1961) theory is probably the best known self theory. He views behaviour as the result of the experience of immediate perceptual events. It is the individual who has the greatest potential for awareness of his own reality. Perceptions are determinants of action in this schema. Rogers argues that the person should be seen as a whole and not broken down into various parts. The central source of personal energy is self-actualisation (see discussion of Maslow in Chapter 9). This is such an all-embracing view of life forces, that motivation can be seen only as an integral part of being alive.

The central concept in Rogers' theory is the self. He characterises this as an organised, consistent amalgam of perceptions of the characteristics of 'I' and of the relations of 'I' to others and to life in general; plus the positive or negative values of these perceptions. Also, through social interaction some of the individual's perceptual field is differentiated into self. The way the individual interprets his self (for example, as weak or strong) affects his perceptions of the rest of the world. The values put into these interpretations can come from direct experience or can be taken from other people.

Rogers suggests that the personality is made up of two systems — the self concept and the organism — which may be opposed or in harmony. If they are opposed, maladjustment may result. If the individual has experiences which are inconsistent with the self they may be perceived as threats. The more such threats there are, the more rigid and defensive becomes the structure of the self and hence the personality. This will lead to a loss of contact with actual experiences.

Also, Rogers suggests that there is a universal need for *positive regard*. All of us desire love and acceptance, both from others and from the self. A genuine adjustment would come from an unconditional positive regard, but of course life is rarely like this. Experiences are sought out or avoided because they are more or less worthy of regard. Any incongruities in this system produce strain which can end in maladjustment. For example, this might be seen in a student who experiences himself as unhappy in his studies but who also sees himself as having to succeed.

This is enough to give the main ideas of Rogers' theory. It typifies phenomenological self theories and has led Rogers to develop the very influential *client-centred therapy* for maladjusted personalities. The aim of this is to achieve a harmonious interaction between the self and the organism and a better congruence between the way the self is structured and the form of an individual's experiences.

The Self: 2 Kelly

Although Kelly's (1955) theory of personality is not strictly a self theory it is sufficiently important and in a similar tradition to that of Rogers to be included here. He argues that the only way to study per-sonality is not to form hypotheses as a scientist but to determine what are the individual's own hypotheses about himself and the world. He views man as a hypothesis creator and a player of roles. Man sets up ideas and dimensions for himself in order to categorise his own exper-iences. To assess his personality the psychologist must pay attention to these rather than to his own views. Kelly argues that all people are alike in constructing hypotheses to understand and control the events in their lives. Hence, in order to understand a person it is necessary to explore his *own* private personality theory.

Of course, a person or persons can construe the same event in many different ways. For example, a young boy hits his father; what does this mean? There are many answers to this, ranging from sheer rage, through accident, to practising his boxing. How it is construed will depend on the individual's viewpoint. Such an idea leads to Kelly's fundamental postulate: 'A person's processes are psychologically channelized by the way in which he anticipates events.' The emphasis is clearly on the sub-jective. Kelly's theory although expressed in great detail, hinges on this fundamental postulate and on a number of similarly stated corollaries into which there is no need to go here.

To Kelly the truth of a person's construct is of secondary impor-tance; of primary importance is its *convenience* to its holder. For example, whether or not a person is highly anxious or highly aggressive, is it convenient for him to construe himself as so being? If not, what would be a more expedient hypothesis for him to hold? Also, Kelly does not view personality as consisting of stable, enduring traits, but rather sees a person as capable of enacting many roles. Without realising it, the individual seems to be attempting to understand someone else through role playing within what he thinks are that person's constructs.

As mentioned above, there are many theories which emphasise the experiential, the subjective, or the self. They reflect an approach to personality which has become relatively popular during the last few years. However, there are criticisms which can be brought to bear on such theories.
(1) Those who are committed to determinism ask, for example, what *causes* a person to self-actualise or to perceive the self in a particular way; questions which it is very difficult for Rogers or Kelly to answer.
(2) It is only an *assumption* (which may be unwarranted) that cogni-

tions or subjective experiences cause behaviour. As far as can be seen the relationship between personal concepts and behaviour is often remote and indirect. There is no certain evidence that cognitive change produces significant behaviour change; on occasion it is even the other way about.

(3) The self and experiential theories of personality are often incomplete. They make no detailed analysis of causes.

(4) The final and most important comment concerns the nature of concepts such as the self. Since it is a descriptive rather than an explanatory concept, it leaves many questions unanswered. For example: is the self a causal agent, making us do things? Is it simply an experienced phenomenon? Is it both of these? If the self does things, what causes it to? Is there another self which controls the first self? Where is the self? Is it tangible? Is it separate from the rest (whatever this might be) of the individual? And so on.

Social-cultural

Whiting and Child (1953) put forward a rather vaguely expressed theory of personality via descriptive comparisons of the way in which the customs of various cultures and societies affect personality and behaviour. They propose a firm relationship between what an individual learns and whatever typifies his culture. For the most part, children learn to behave in ways which are approved by adults, but the patterns of what is approved are quite distinctive in different cultures. To Whiting and Child culture is an important determinant of personality.

As will be seen later, socialisation is always concerned with changing the behaviour patterns of a child into those of an adult. As Whiting and Child see it, infants exist in a period of indulgence and then later are forced to modify their behaviour and hence their personalities into society's norms. The point in time at which this happens differs from society to society and has different social procedures to bring it about. All of this has its effects on personality. For example, there are some societies in which there is not time of adolescence as we know it in western society. An individual passes from childhood to adulthood within a few weeks or even days — with some ceremonies to mark the passage. This must make clear differences to personality. In their analysis, Whiting and Child lay particular emphasis on the effects on personality of differences in the age at which weaning occurs and the style in which it is accomplished.

A more specific example of this type of approach to personality comes from the work of Adorno et al (1950) on the *authoritarian* personality. They lay stress on the influence of family and parental discipline on the development of personality. Their research, questionable though it is in some ways, points to the authoritarian personality characterising a person who has had a highly protected upbringing. The authoritarian believes the world to be a dangerous place in which children should be obedient to their parents. Any transgressions should be severely punished. As children they tend to have experienced severe discipline themselves but to have repressed any hostile feelings they might have had towards their parents. Also they tend to deny any basic aggressive or sexual feelings they might experience.

These ideas on a particular type of personality are just one example of the many attempts which have been made to relate personality to upbringing and type of parental discipline. As might be imagined, the evidence for such theories is somewhat shaky because it is almost always retrospective. People who are assessed as having particular personality characteristics are asked questions about their childhood and family experiences. Their answers are inevitably open to any manner of distortion and error. It would be hopelessly uneconomic (in both time and money) to carry out longitudinal studies tracing personality development throughout the lives of a group of people and relating it to their upbringing, whilst trying to assess the influence of all the other possible determinants.

Stimulus-response

Stimulus-response or social behavioural theories of personality are best exemplified by the ideas of Dollard and Miller (1950), Bandura and Walters (1963) and Gewirtz (1969). Behavioural theories of personality dwell on what the individual is doing and renounce what they believe to be the vaguer notions of other theories, such as motive and traits; and they ignore concepts such as the content of human nature. As ever, they argue that it is impossible to characterise man as apart from his environment. The aim of S-R theories of personality is to clarify conditions that control behaviour, and hence personality. They attempt to make specific causal analyses of personality.

Oddly enough, S-R theories are similar to psychoanalytic theories in that they place great importance on the first five years of life. However, rather than making personality dependent on hidden dynamic forces, they suggest that it is determined by specific patterns of reinforcement. The argument is that the child is born with a built-in hierarchy of responses which controls the order in which responses might be made to specific situations. It may be for example that at a certain stage a child is set to respond more immediately to food than to people.

The general development of personality is seen as occurring through a series of learning processes which depend on external reinforcement. Again, the processes involved may be very similar to those mentioned in psychoanalytic theory; weaning, toilet training, and so on. The reinforcement will be selective of certain responses and the learning may very well be happening at a subconscious level.

Probably the single most important detail of S-R theories of personality is that the mother is regarded as a secondary reinforcer. She acquires this status because of her constant association with the primary, built-in reinforcers of food and warmth. Through this association, the child's mother is able herself to reinforce new learning and so exercise control over the developing personality. This is a very steady, gradual process of learning which is helped along by generalisation. Since the child learns to respond in particular ways through the reinforcing power of its mother, and because other people are like her, then similar responses will be made to them, and so personality develops in relation to other people. The whole process moves onto an even broader footing when the child branches out from the home into school life.

In general, S-R theory of personality has it that learning is at the basis of personality and that learning is influenced by the situation in which it occurs and/or by the reinforcers which promote it. The strength of this type of theory is that it rejects rather unwieldy constructs such as ego or self, and aims at descriptions which are as specific as possible. The study of personality becomes an analysis of behavioural change. Of course, it can be argued that this is a debasing of personality, and that personality is clearly more than just behaviour. The S-R approach does see personality as fragmentary, does not allow for integration, and views humans as rather passive. And it may well be that other types of personality theorist are right to insist that in this case the whole is greater than the sum of the parts and that personality can only be understood if man is viewed as a complete integrated whole, behaviour being but one small part of this.

Psychometrics

As the name implies, psychometrics is concerned with *measurement* of personality. However, the psychometric approach has led not only to the construction of measurement techniques but also to the development of theories of personality. It is an approach which is centred on the *organisation* of personality, which it assumes is built round a set of basic traits or characteristics, identified by complex statistical techniques. Essentially, the psychometric approach to personality theory dwells on *description* and has little to say of development. The usual assumption is that personality traits develop through a mixture of childhood experiences and built-in propensities.

A good introduction to psychometric theory can be found in Cattell (1965) who has done more in this area than anyone else. He has a complex descriptive theory which revolves round personality being made up of 16 basic traits. However, for present purposes it is more appropriate to describe the rather simpler theory of Eysenck (e.g. 1953).

For many years Eysenck argued that personality is made up of two fundamental traits, which we all have in some degree. 1) Neuroticism, which is akin to anxiety, and 2) Extroversion/introversion, which can be roughly described as the degree to which a person is outgoing or turned inwards. Eysenck's many hundreds of studies all point to these characteristics being at the basis of whatever other traits develop later, and that they in turn depend on inherited propensities in the nervous system which are compounded by life experiences.

In technical terms, Eysenck describes these two dimensions as orthogonal, that is they are entirely unrelated (at right angles graphically) to each other. They can be most easily expressed in diagrammatic form. Any individual has a place on this diagram. Thus for example if a man were highly extroverted and of low neuroticism, he would appear in the bottom left hand corner. Whereas, if he were of average neuroticism and fairly introverted, he would appear on the E/I line towards the I end. Eysenck has devised personality scales (of good reliability and validity) in order to measure these two dimensions. Latterly, Eysenck (1976) has added a third orthogonal dimension to these two, psychoticism, although the evidence for this is not yet as clear as for the other two.

In summary, the psychometric approach to personality is concerned with describing personality by identifying basic personality traits. This means that it is nicely quantifiable and measurable and as such might be said to be better than many other theories. On the other hand, such theories make certain assumptions which must still be regarded as arbitrary and therefore open to question. For example, do a finite number of personality traits exist? If they do, all well and good; if not, the psychometric approach becomes hopelessly unwieldy. Is each trait a continuum on which any person has his place? If not, then again confusion will develop. And finally, are all traits independent? The evidence on this is very shaky, particularly when a theory, like Cattell's, contains as many as 16 traits.

Finally, the most telling criticism of trait theory as it is sometimes called, is that those who adhere to it sometimes forget that it is essentially *descriptive*, and attempt to use traits in *explanatory* ways. This is both unjustified and unhelpful. For example, assume that one basic trait is dominance and then anyone can be assessed as to his degree of dominance. This is acceptable descriptively. Now imagine that a person who has a measured high dominance score is seen to dominate a social gathering. The question 'why' is asked and the answer given 'because he is dominant'. At the every-day level this type of answer is often accepted, but it is nonsense. It merely re-describes the behaviour; it does not explain it. Of course, this criticism is not really of trait or psychometric theory, but of the rather poor way in which it is sometimes extended.

Conclusions

As was stated in the introduction to this chapter, there are many theories of personality. The aim here has been to describe some of the more influential of these and in so doing give some idea of the various approaches which they reflect. A far more complete overview can be found in Hall and Lindzey (1970). At present no one of these theories or even approaches has gained general acceptance. Freudian theory dominated interest for many years, but it has obvious shortcomings of untestability and unpredictability. To some extent it was replaced by the S-R approach with its emphasis on social behaviourism, but this rather does away with personality and replaces it with behaviour and reinforcement; an approach which is not to some people's taste, particularly if they believe that personality exists in its own right and has a causal role to play in human functioning. More recently the self-oriented phenomenological theories of psychologists such as Rogers and Kelly have received much attention, since they reflect the humanist (anti-behaviourist) movement in psychology (particularly American psychology). But again, they leave many questions unanswered, especially concerning the nature and status of 'self'.

Perhaps the main problem with the study of personality is that like many aspects of psychology it hinges on a word which is in common everyday use and which has a large number of connotations at this level. Doubtless, many of these connotations have influenced and perhaps biassed the work of those psychologists who have become interested in it. Unfortunately however, in spite of the large amount of work done, the word personality has not yet received a substantive and generally agreed meaning within academic psychology. Ultimately, it may be that it is found to be a not very helpful concept in predicting and explaining human endeavours. Or if it is then this is only at a relatively mundane level.

Of course, there are good academic and practical reasons for studying personality, but the main reason of all is in order to make predictions about what an *individual* will do; to predict individual behaviour. As can be seen throughout this book, most of psychology's predictions are statistical or actuarial; given conditions a, b, and c then 95 from a 100 people with characteristics and experiences x, y and z will go left rather than right. But the ultimate aim is to predict what a given individual will do under any circumstances. Personality is the main area of study in which the individual is investigated as a fully integrated whole rather than being analysed into his parts and lumped together with others.

The basic assumption is that established patterns of behaviour *will* recur and that these recurrences can be predicted from a knowledge of the individual personality. Although this seems a reasonable assumption, none of the approaches to personality theory described above actually deal with *situations* in which behaviour occurs (with the possible exception of S-R theory). In order to make accurate predictions such an approach would be necessary. For example, assume that a person has been reliably assessed as shy and another as anxious. One needs to be able to predict *when* the shyness or anxiety will show itself, and under what *conditions*. In order to do this it is necessary to study the individuals in specific situations. Even if a personality theory is so good as to provide accurate descriptions and measurements, the characteristics it finds in an individual case will only show themselves under some conditions and at some times. It is this information which is required for individual prediction. If a person is a highly introverted neurotic he is not *always* in the same state. Why not? What causes the changes? As yet personality theory cannot answer these questions.

Summary Points

(1) The study of personality involves the investigation of the whole person over time. When this is done, his behaviour seems to be consistent, organised and unique. Research into personality has revolved round the many definitions and theories which have been proposed.
(2) The best known constitutional theory of personality is Sheldon's who attempted to link body type with personality type, his categories of these being endomorphy (viscerotonic), mesomorphy (somatotonic) and ectomorphy (cerebrotonic).

(3) The most influential theory of personality has been that of Freud who couched it in terms of three mental energy systems, the id, ego and superego. It is a developmental theory, with stress being laid on early developmental problems providing prototypical personality patterns for the potential adult. Freud centred interest on the three erotogenic areas of the body, the mouth, the anus and the genitalia, in children up to the age of five. This type of approach has been carried on by neo-Freudians.

(4) Self theories of personality represent a recent upsurge of interest in the phenomenological approach to psychology. They are well exemplified by Rogers who gives a central role to the self and to the motive of self-actualisation, and by Kelly who believed that to gain an understanding of man it is necessary to find out how he conceptualises himself and the world.

(5) Socio-cultural theories of personality emphasise early environmental influences on the developing personality. They stress cultural differences in weaning and early upbringing.

(6) Stimulus-response theories of personality lay stress on the development of social behaviour through selective reinforcement. Personality becomes little more than behaviour and develops through the individual interacting with his environment.

(7) Psychometric theories of personality depend on a belief that personality is made up of a series of traits on which people are comparable. The main exponents of these theories are Cattell with his 16 factors and Eysenck with neuroticism and extroversion/introversion. They are descriptive rather than explanatory theories.

(8) The study of personality and the struggle to provide an adequate theory of personality has been bedevilled by the fact that personality is a word with a rich variety of everyday meanings. Particular difficulty comes with the main aim of work in this area which is to make individual predictions. Most personality theories do not permit this since they are not concerned with looking at the individual in particular situations. Personality characteristics might be enduring and relatively stable, but they are not constant. To make precise predictions it is necessary to determine what an individual of personality x will do in situation y at time z.

Study Questions – 10

(1) Of the personality theories you have studied, which do you think is of most help in understanding the personalities of the people with whom you come into contact professionally? Why?

(2) Have you ever seen any striking changes of personality in a patient during the course of his treatment or therapy? What do you think caused them?

(3) In your judgement, do illness, injury, or hospitalisation bring about changes in personality? Do you think that such changes would be lasting?

(4) Freudian theory is very much concerned with the underlying motivations and dynamics of personality. Are such concerns of any importance to you in the routine of your professional endeavours? Do they help you to understand your patients?

(5) Have you found that some personalities are better able to withstand accident and injury than others? What characterises such personalities?

(6) Do you think that some personalities are more suitable for training in the paramedical services than others? What characterises such personalities?

(7) Attempt to write full descriptions of the personalities of three people who have had very different types of disability or disease. Do you think that type of disease or disability and personality are related?

(8) What do you think are the main influences on personality? Has your personality been changed at all by anything you have experienced during your training?

(9) Attempt to see if there are any points in common amongst the personalities of the most difficult and recalcitrant patients with whom you have had to deal. What can you do about a patient whose personality seems to be persistently negative?

(10) What is your reaction to the attitude that 'people are people', that all illness and injury are sheerly medical matters, and hence that personality and individual differences in reactions should be of little importance to members of the paramedical professions.

11 INTELLIGENCE

Definitions

Just as with personality, there have been numerous definitions of intelligence and there is still no consensus of opinion as to which of them is the most appropriate. It is one of those words about which almost everybody, psychologist and non-psychologist alike, has something to say. In the early history of research into intelligence, there were two types of definition, each with its limitations. (1) Intelligence is the degree to which a person can adapt to fresh situations; a definition so broad as to be of limited use. (2) Intelligence is what the intelligence tests measure; which, ducking the issue, is hardly a definition at all. As is so often the case, in reaction to these limitations, more recent definitions have been a compromise. Briefly these suggest that intelligence is an *inferred attribute which is relatively long lasting and which is concerned with an individual's ability to react successfully to a variety of problems and circumstances.*

There has also grown up a tradition of dividing intelligence into two aspects. This began with Hebb (1949) who suggested that there is intelligence A and intelligence B. Intelligence A is the *innate potential* with which we are born and which sets the limits on any development. This potential cannot be measured. Intelligence B is what we have achieved, influenced by the environment, and is what is measured by intelligence tests. From this viewpoint an intelligence test only gives an assessment of what an individual has achieved and not of what he might be potentially capable given different circumstances.

It is impossible to observe intelligence; it is an inferred capacity. However, it is possible to observe people taking tests designed to measure intelligence and to collect their scores. When such tests have been standardised, it is possible to derive from their scores an indication of *mental age* and to transform this into an *intelligence quotient* (IQ) for the individual. This is given by the simple formula:

$$IQ = \frac{MA}{CA} \times 100$$

Given the way they are derived IQs are normally distributed (statistically speaking) in the overall population, around a mean of 100. Just as with psychometric tests of personality, intelligence tests and measures of IQ provide a reference point to make comparisons between people. They are relative rather than absolute.

The Structure of Intelligence

Intelligence was the first enduring trait to be measured and more recently has been the trait which is most frequently measured. In the past most intelligence tests were designed in the belief that they would be concerned with a single, unitary concept. However, more recently, psychologists have argued against this and have suggested instead that intelligence is made up of many different aspects which might even be unrelated within one individual.

There are three main exponents of this view. (1) Thurstone (1938) concluded from his studies that there are nine primary mental abilities. These are: word fluency, verbal ability, induction, deduction, reasoning ability, spatial ability, numerical ability, perceptual speed, and rote memory. He argued that these abilities are so independent of one another as to be incapable of grouping into a single meaningful score.

(2) Spearman (1927) by contrast believed that the main aspect of intelligence is a huge *general factor* (g) which underpins all forms that intelligence might take. Although he felt that it should be the main aim of intelligence tests to measure this g factor, he also believed there to be a number of *specific factors* which determine special abilities and which only make their contribution in specific situations, adding some complexity to g.

(3) Guilford (1967). More recently, Guilford has suggested that there are 120 factors which make up intelligence. These came from combinations of three dimensions of intellectual performance: a) operations, b) contents, and c) products. He argues that his own research has already proved the existence of 100 of these factors.

Ultimately of course, the measurement of intelligence is a highly practical matter aimed at practical utility. So, even if Guilford is correct his ideas have limited application in a practical world. There must be more simplification if the aim is to provide a measure of intelligence which can be taken fairly rapidly and used straight away. Also, the problem still remains as to whether intelligence is made up of a general factor *plus* specific abilities, or is just a conglomeration of specific capacities.

Characteristics of IQ

IQ is the normally accepted reflection of intelligence. It is therefore important to describe its characteristics.

(1) Short-term change

Over brief periods of time in the individual case, IQs change very little, unless of course there are extreme changes in the environment. Put another way, this means that there is high test-retest reliability in the standard intelligence tests.

(2) Long-term change

In spite of the relative absence of IQ change in the short term, IQs do alter systematically with time. It seems that there are changes in the *rate* of intellectual development. Some children change very little and others very much, depending on their environment. However, it is very difficult to predict these changes since it is virtually impossible to determine IQ in an infant and so to establish a baseline from which to work.

(3) Old age

As will be seen in later chapters, there are two major ways of studying development; by investigating samples of people of various ages (cross-section) and by investigating one group of people over a long period of time (longitudinal). These two approaches give opposed findings with respect to IQ changes in the old. The cross-sectional method suggests that IQ deteriorates in the old, particularly when the test is concerned with novel situations. However, longitudinal studies suggest that there is no IQ decline throughout middle age, although there is some falling off after this.

At present, it is impossible to say which of these two results is correct. There are many problems. For example, studying cross-sections of people does not allow proper comparisons to be made, with respect to intelligence, since the educational experiences and opportunities of the people in the various groups will have been different. On the other hand, when studying one group over a long time it is inevitable that some subjects are lost; they die, move away, or otherwise cannot be contacted. Such losses *might* introduce a systematic bias into results.

(4) The extremes

Mental retardation is difficult to define and to say where mental retardation begins and ends. Suffice it to say that it describes those individuals who have very low IQs, 69 points at the most. There are various levels of mental retardation which are described below, although these cannot be tied exactly to particular IQ ranges. Whether or not the mentally retarded can ever achieve normal adjustment depends on many factors other than their basic IQ.

It is clear that there are some extreme consequences to behaviour of very low IQs. However, it should be borne in mind that some of these results are not inevitable. They are due to people's expectations. If people are told that an individual they are to meet has a very low IQ, then they will have certain vague expectations about him, and these expectations might well push the individual further in that direction. This is simply the usual way in which stereotypes work.

(a) The *mildly* retarded are generally slow to mature and in some cases might not be noticed as retarded at all. They can be trained in practical skills and can be taught simple reading and arithmetic, and can be guided into relatively normal social behaviour. As adults they can maintain themselves, socially and emotionally, but need support when they are stressed.

(b) The *moderately* retarded show some delays in their motor development, particularly in speech. They can be trained in simple communications and to learn health and safety rules, and some manual skills. As adults they can perform simple tasks in sheltered workshops, and can enjoy simple relaxation, but they cannot fully maintain themselves.

(c) The *severely* retarded have great delays in their motor development, have virtually no communication abilities but can be taught to feed themselves. They can usually walk and have very simple habits trained. As adults they need constant supervision and protection and do little other than the most simple repetitive routines.

(d) The *profoundly* retarded show enormous retardation, need to be nursed constantly, and have only the very minimum of human capacities. They can never maintain themselves in any way at all, and only in very rare cases will ever walk or speak. Training is almost impossible.

It is important to realise that most cases of mental retardation are *not* the result of any obvious structural problems, although some relatively rare cases are — for example phenylketonuria (6 in 100,000) and Down's syndrome (mongolism) which results from an extra chromosome at conception and occurs at the high rate of 1 in 60 children born to mothers who are 45 plus. However, it seems that many mental retardates have simply not had the opportunities to learn. Changes in the environment should reverse this in some cases and enable the individual to come a little nearer to realising his innate potential.

Gifted individuals are at the other end of the IQ range, the normal cut-off point for defining gifted being taken as 140 or more IQ points. However, IQs considerably in excess of this have been *estimated* (it is difficult to assess them) perhaps going as high as 190 or 200. At present, unfortunately, little can be said about gifted people since they have been relatively neglected both in research and in practice. It is to be hoped that this state of affairs is changing.

IQ and other aspects of performance

One of the basic reasons for attempting to measure intelligence has been to try to predict from it to success in various areas of life. Also, many people have been interested in determining the extent to which intelligence contributes to success. To these ends there is a long history of research attempting to relate IQ to other measures of performance.

(1) School performance

There are a large number of studies which show a positive correlation between scholastic attainment and IQ. However, none of these studies demonstrates any causal relationships; they neither show that high IQ leads to high educational attainment or that scholastic success leads to the development of a higher IQ. The basic problem is that many factors other than IQ affect or are related to academic merit; motivation, perseverance, self-confidence, and so on. This means that some people with high IQs do only averagely well at school, and some of those of average IQ do very well.

It is certainly the case that IQs predict school performance *better* than does anything else, but they allow far from perfect predictions and should never therefore be used alone. The problem is that not all tests on which IQs are based correlate equally well with school performance and it is by no means certain that scholastic success is exactly measured by school examinations.

(2) Occupation

Much use is made of IQ in selecting people for jobs, it being crudely believed that the higher a person's IQ the more likely he is to do well in a given occupation and the more capable he will be of success in the more demanding occupations. Again, the relationship between occupation and IQ is not as straightforward as might be expected. Some occupations do demand higher IQs; this is obvious. You need to be brighter to fly a modern jet aircraft than to sweep up a road. Also, in general, occupations of greater prestige than average contain more people with relatively high IQs than those with low prestige. However, once again, no statements can be made about the direction of any causal relationships. Do more intelligent people seek out more demanding, high prestige jobs, or do such jobs promote more intelligent behaviour, or both?

(3) General Success

Are those people with relatively high IQs also happier and more successful than the average? Fincher (1973) made a full analysis of this question, basing it largely on a follow up of Terman's work carried out many years previously. Terman undertook a longitudinal study on approximately 1,500 American children with IQs of 140 plus. In comparison with their contemporaries, he found them to be heavier at birth, taller as adults, constantly ahead at school, gravitating to leadership, very successful and with relatively few aspects of their lives going wrong.

On the face of it, it would seem that high IQ does lead to relatively great general success and hence happiness, if the two can be equated. However, once again there are caveats. Does all this general success in life come about through high IQ or through a more stimulating family background, which might also promote high IQ? Why did not *all* the people studied by Terman achieve general success? Many did not who were as bright as those who did. Clearly then, a high IQ does not guarantee general success in life; there are many other factors which have an influence. And of course for the same reason general success does not guarantee happiness.

(4) Creativity

As has been seen at other points in this book, creativity is a very difficult topic to investigate and the relationship between IQ and creativity is problematic. However, at this point it is worth summarising the conclusions drawn by Gough (1964) on this topic. There *may* very well be differences between the person who is highly intelligent in the conventional sense and the person who is highly creative. However, in general, Gough suggests that the creative individual: (a) differs little in intelligence from anyone else, (b) he thinks flexibly, (c) he has uncommon perceptions and associations, (d) he is not much concerned with accuracy but dwells on form, (e) he is intuitive and empathetic being interested for example in *why* people do things rather than how, (f) he is open to novel ideas, (g) he is sensitive, and (h) it almost goes without saying, he has a complex personality. The relationship between IQ and creativity is unclear, although it is true to say that Gough's description is not of a high IQ person, necessarily. Whether or not creativity is a necessary part of intelligence or intelligence a necessary part of creativity remains to be seen.

Intelligence and Background: The Nature/Nurture Question

Throughout the history of its assessment there has been fierce controversy concerning the relative contributions made to intelligence by heredity and environment. In the early days this took the form of an expert in one or other camp making a strong avowal that intelligence is, say 80 per cent heredity and 20 per cent environment, or 80 per cent environment and 20 per cent heredity. After some years the sterility of this debate was realised and a more enlightened position arrived at; namely, that intelligence is determined by an interaction between nature and nurture which is so complex as to render it both impossible and meaningless to try to assign proportional degrees of influence to them.

Throughout these skirmishes between the hereditarians and environmentalists a great deal of research was done which bears on the question. It is important to describe some of this and its attendant problems. This is not only in an attempt to be comprehensive but also because the heredity/environment question has recently flared up again in relation to intelligence and race. It is necessary to set the record as straight as it can be about such an emotive issue.

Family and Twin Studies

One way in which attempts have been made to assess the influence of heredity on intelligence is to compare the IQs of various members of families, i.e. between parents and children and between siblings. When this is done the positive correlations which describe the patterns are found to approach 0.5 which is quite large, similar correlations being found in families for physical dimensions such as height. However, it is impossible to draw any conclusion from studies such as this. Is the similarity in IQ due to similar genetic make-up or to the shared environment that most families enjoy? One could get nearer to this question if it were possible to test intelligence at birth, but this cannot be done.

These difficulties led to the study of adopted children. Do their IQs resemble more closely those of their real (biological) parents or those of their adoptive parents? There are two answers to this question. First, the correlations in IQ between adopted children and their *real* parents are higher than those with their adoptive parents: a genetic influence.

Second, in spite of this, the IQs of adopted children tend to be higher than would be predicted by extrapolation from the IQs of their real parents. The correlation is positive but the children's IQs seem to have been shifted up en masse. This is thought to be due to the *generally* favourable atmosphere of adoptive homes, one of the bases on which they are chosen: an environmental influence.

Ideally, in order to study the heredity/environment question, it would be appropriate to hold one constant whilst varying the other. Of course this is impossible to do with environment, it cannot be held constant. No two people can be in the same place at the same time; no two people have ever had or can ever have the same environment. However it can occur with heredity. Identical (monozygotic) twins have *exactly* the same genetic make-up since they result from the splitting of a fertilised egg. By contrast, fraternal twins (dizygotic) result from the near simultaneous fertilisation of two eggs and hence have genetic structures as similar as those of ordinary siblings, although they do of course share a very *similar* environment from conception onwards.

Twin studies concerning intelligence have led to a number of well-established findings.
(1) Identical twins rarely have identical IQs, but the differences between them are usually less than 10 points; they are very similar.
(2) Fraternal twins are less similar in IQ than identical twins but still a little more similar than ordinary siblings.
(3) The IQs of identical twins separated at birth and raised in different families (something which has happened surprisingly often over the years) are less similar than those of identical twins brought up together.

Once again then, such studies do not allow the precise sorting out of the nature/nurture question. As the various comparisons of IQ are made so the findings point first to genetic influence and then immediately to environmental influences.

Social Class

In the early history of research into intelligence there were several studies which showed that in general people who live in cities had higher IQs than those that live in rural areas. This was thought by some to support a heredity argument and by others to support an environmentalist position. Of course, once again, it is impossible to separate the two. It may be that in the days when such differences were observed, brighter people migrated to towns because they had the numerical and language skills that city life tends to require, or alternatively it may be that the generally more stimulating (in some ways) life in towns and cities brought about improvements in IQ.

This leads onto the important work of Sir Cyril Burt who was much concerned with the nature/nurture problem in intelligence. Here is not the place to review Burt's very large contribution, but it is important to give an idea of the type of study he made and the type of conclusions which he drew.

In 1961 Burt compared the IQs of large numbers of London school children and their parents. He divided them into six socio-economic classes on the basis of parental occupation. His main findings were:
(1) The average IQs of parents were closely related to socio-economic class.
(2) Within any one class there was large variation in parental IQ.
(3) The variability in the children's IQs was the same as that in the general population.
(4) The average IQs of children within a class was halfway between the average IQ of the parents in that class and the overall population average of 100. So, if the average parental IQ was 120, the average child IQ in that class was 110; if the parental IQ was 90, the child average was 95.

On the basis of these and other results, Burt concluded that IQ is an important determinant of occupational class and that it is *appreciably* inherited. These conclusions were perhaps not entirely justified, but Burt was anyway a great believer in genetic influences. As an aside, Burt also concluded that it is important that there be mobility between classes if what is technically termed regression to the mean is to be counteracted. That is, if there were not class mobility then successive generations would end up closer and closer to the population mean IQ of 100, and everyone would eventually be of average intelligence, which fortunately does not happen.

Race

Strictly speaking, human races are subgroups within a species. Over long periods of time it is assumed that people remaining in localised groups plus natural selection (in the Darwinian sense) has produced group differences, which in turn become maintained and reinforced by cultural differentiation. Some racial differences obviously have a genetic origin, skin colour being the most evident example. (Although it is worth noting that even with skin colour temporary changes can be effected environmentally; people do so on beaches every summer.) However, the most important question concerns whether or not complex behaviour such as that which is involved in intelligence has a sufficient genetic component to lead to racial differences.

Much of the research bearing on this matter has been conducted in the USA where comparisons have been made between the IQs of blacks and whites. The general finding has been that on average the IQs of whites are higher than those of blacks; not only is this true but also in specific regions of the USA. However, there is considerable overlap between the two groups. This potentially inflammatory difference was raised with some force by Jensen (1969) who assesses the evidence as demonstrating that the measured differences in IQ between blacks and whites might well be determined *to some extent* by genetic factors. Certainly, from some viewpoints such differences look to have a genetic basis, particularly when one considers that they persist within a single socio-economic level where there is reasonable similarity between possible environmental influences such as education, occupation and income.

There are however many reasons why Jensen's arguments do not stand up to scrutiny, or at least can be seen as premature. The list that follows is taken mainly from a cogent analysis and review made by Bodmer and Cavalli-Sforza (1970).

(1) Even within one socio-economic level how can the statuses of blacks and whites be compared? Black schools are poorer, black occupations are worse (within any one level), and there are 200 years of prejudice, the influences of which cannot be forgotten. Overall, *matching* is impossible.

(2) There is a vast *variation* in IQ within the white population.

(3) Most IQ tests are given by middle class whites and one of the aspects of giving a test is to obtain a representative sample of behaviour by establishing a proper *rapport* with the testee. This would be more difficult to establish between white and black, particularly if they are of different social classes, than between two people of the same colour and class. In fact the IQs of blacks tested by whites are on average two to three points lower than when they are tested by other blacks.

(4) It is established that IQ is related to diet and its deficiencies. In general, blacks have poorer diets than whites.

(5) The early home environment is known to be important in the development of intelligence. In general, that of blacks is poorer than that of whites.

(6) It is well established in psychology that if someone expects to fail or to do poorly at something then this will be more likely to happen than if he thinks he will be successful. Given their living conditions and poor opportunities, blacks will feel themselves to do poorly at anything, including intelligence tests, than whites.

Bodmer and Cavalli-Sforza conclude, as do many other investigators, that there is no hard and fast evidence to support Jensen's contentions. Properly to test the question of racial differences in IQ there would need to be large numbers of properly controlled studies, which, given the complexities discussed above, would be impossible to run. There *may* be genetic differences between blacks and whites but there is no reason to suppose that the genes which affect intelligence should be such as to differ between races.

Conclusions

Since there has been so much public interest in the assessment of intelligence there have been many misconceptions about it. A long tradition of research has given the lie to these. For example, it is *wrong* to think that:
(1) intelligence is inherited,
(2) mental ability does not increase after 13,
(3) high IQ guarantees high achievement,
(4) people with high IQs are likely to be disturbed emotionally,
(5) blonds have lower IQs than brunettes,
(6) males or females are brighter than females or males,
(7) sportsmen have low IQs,
(8) anyone is intelligent enough to do anything given the opportunity,
(9) low IQ people are strong and high IQ people are weak.
All of these statements are more incorrect than correct.

Although intelligence testing has a very long history, nowadays society seems to be beginning to place values on qualities other than intelligence. For example, there is more and more talk of allowing people to lead more creative, fulfilled and self-actualised lives, and to give them equal opportunities to do so. Although it is sometimes useful to test IQs in order to make predictions about people's capabilities, to saddle them with some descriptive label on the basis of such testing may very well lead to self-fulfilling prophecies and to put such people under considerable pressure. The low IQ person may sink even lower, and the high IQ person may feel constant pressure to demonstrate his worth.

It is perhaps worth saying a final word about the matter of heredity/ environment and intelligence, particularly as it pertains to race. Overall, it can be argued on three main grounds that it would be better to undertake less of this type of research. First, most psychologists recognise that intelligence is contributed to by a complex interaction between genetic and environmental influences and it is therefore not worth trying to separate their effects. Second, studies on race and IQ would not throw much light on the genetic control of IQ; there are more cogent studies which could be made out of this. Finally, if equal opportunities are of concern, it is individual rather than racial differences that should be considered. As studies and ideas such as Jensen's could easily be misinterpreted by racists, they are perhaps better left undone.

Summary Points

(1) Intelligence has been defined in many ways, none of which is fully satisfactory, and concern with its assessment has led to the development of the IQ as a comparative measure.

(2) Many early tests treated intelligence as a unitary concept but more recent ones have seen it as a mixture of many specific abilities. It is still impossible to decide whether or not there is a general factor in intelligence as Spearman suggested.

(3) Measured IQs have a number of characteristics. Over short periods of time they remain fairly constant but over long periods they can change. The evidence on what happens to IQs in later life remains equivocal. There has been a great deal of work on the mentally retarded, although much less on those with very high IQs.

(4) IQ is related to both scholastic and occupational success, but since the data are only correlational, no statements can be made about casual connections. Also, high IQ does not guarantee success and IQ is not necessarily related to creativity.

(5) The nature/nurture question in intelligence has long been of concern. Evidence from family studies, twin studies, and studies on social class point to a complex interaction between the two. Such studies reach their peak in the matter of racial differences in intelligence, particularly with respect to black and white Americans. The present evidence can point in a number of directions and the general conclusion is that there are so many complicated environmental influences that cannot be properly controlled, it is impossible to assess the influence of heredity at all precisely.

(6) The future of intelligence testing is perhaps in the balance. Recently, society seems to emphasising other aspects of human functioning.

Study Questions – 11

(1) How does the intelligence of a patient alter your reactions to him?

Do you think that your behaviour *has* to alter towards patients as a function of their intelligence? If so, in what ways must you take it into account?

(2) In your dealings with patients and colleagues have you seen more than one type of intelligence? If so, what are the characteristics of the main types you have seen?

(3) Would it help you in your job if at some appropriate time each of your patients were given an intelligence test? Do you think that the results of such a test given in a hospital would be at all representative?

(4) What would be the differences in your approach to a highly intelligent but unmotivated patient and a highly motivated but very unintelligent patient?

(5) Have you ever observed what you would consider to be racial and cultural differences in intelligence? If so, what do you think brings them about?

(6) In your role in helping a patient to recover from illness or adjust to disability, what do you consider to be more important, his motivation, his personality, or his intelligence?

(7) How important a part has been played by intelligence in your own training? What has been the relationship between intelligence and creativity in your training?

(8) Do you think that the fairly extreme experiences that some of your patients must have had could lead to permanent alterations in their intelligence (brain-damaged cases apart).

(9) Do people who are at either extreme of the distribution of intelligence react differently to illness or injury? Would you care for them in different ways, using different techniques?

(10) How would you distinguish between intelligence and common-sense? Which of these is the more important in your profession? Why? Have you ever seen any examples of people who are highly intelligent but who lack common-sense, or who have a good share of common-sense but are relatively dull? Which of the two would be the more easily dealt with in a patient?

12 INTERPERSONAL RELATIONSHIPS

Interpersonal relationships are a matter of communication and usually occur and develop without people thinking about them very much. Although in this context communication may be thought to refer to what people say to one another, this is only the obvious part. Certainly, it is very important, but it is not the special concern of this chapter. Here, interest centres on rather more subtle and less obvious aspects of communications that go on between people. Some of these are familiar and some are not, at least until they are pointed out.

At the basis of interpersonal relationships are a series of *rules* which appear to govern how people interact. Again, although they work by these rules, they might not be able to describe them however familiar they might seem to be once they are mentioned. Also, concern centres on what have been termed social *techniques*. To speak of techniques makes the matter of interpersonal relationships seem to be very consciously manipulative, even Machiavellian. Although this sometimes might be so, in the vast majority of interactions, people do not seem to be making conscious attempts to manipulate one another. Be this as it may, there do seem to be great consistencies in the way they use their bodies and eyes for example in communication; these can be employed consciously, and might as well therefore be regarded as techniques.

As will be pointed out in the next chapter, we need as much information as possible to make predictions about what those with whom we interact will shortly be doing. If we were not able to do this, social interactions and interpersonal relationships would be hopelessly out of joint. Probably the most subtle information we use to make such predictions, and to ease social intercourse, comes from the very wide range of intricate variations in communication which will be described later in this chapter.

Status and Solidarity

Two of the most important rules which govern social encounters come from status and solidarity which many social psychologists would argue are at the very basis of interpersonal relationships. The influence of these principles can be seen most clearly in a fascinating analysis of how we address others when we speak to them which is made by Brown (1966).

195

Forms of Address

Typically, in the English language, there is a choice of the form it is
possible to use when addressing others. It is possible to use a person's
first name, or his last name plus his title (Mary, or Miss Smith) and more
rarely it is possible to use the title alone (Doctor) or a nickname (really
an extension of using a first name). Other languages offer rather
more complex alternatives, by having different forms of personal pronoun. Examples come from German (du or sie) and French (tu or vous).
The ways in which these forms of address are used follow rules which
are implicitly understood by those who use them and which therefore
allow predictions to be made about the relationship between the
addressor and the addressee. We would normally assume for example
that there would be a closer, more intimate relationship between two
people who were on first name terms than between those who used last
names plus titles. Also, we would make different assumptions if one
member of a pair used the other's first name and the other used the
former's last name plus title.

In general, where the relationship between two people is one in
which their *status* differences are obvious, what seems to be an *asymmetrical* rule governs the way they address each other. The person of higher
status tends to use the more familiar form of address to his junior and
the person of junior status uses the more distant, more polite form of
address to his senior. So a boss might call his employee by his first
name whereas the employee calls his boss by his last name plus title.

In fact, this status rule has a very long history. For example in
medieval Europe members of the nobility used the more familiar form
of the pronoun (tu or du) when speaking to commoners, whereas
commoners used the more distant form when replying (vous or sie).
Parents gave the more familiar form to their children and received the
more distant form in return. Typically when two people were of equal
status they exchanged the same form of address; the polite form for the
upper classes, and the more familiar form for the lower classes.

It should be obvious from this discussion so far, that the status rule
is not the only one which governs the way in which we address people
today. More commonly now the *solidarity* rule is important. All of us
have some people whose welfare concerns us more than that of other
people; this might be due to similarities in age, kinship, interests or
whatever. We are relatively close to these people. Clearly enough in
addressing such people we would normally use the more intimate form
of address be this first name or the more familiar form of the pronoun
in those languages which permit it. Also, relative strangers use the more

distant form of address.

The two rules or norms of status and solidarity combine to make a two-dimensional system which although quite clear does have its problems.

(1) The more familiar form of address expresses *intimacy* when it is used mutually and *condescension* (talking down) when it is used non-reciprocally.

(2) The more distant form of address expresses *formality* when it is used mutually, and *deference* when used non-reciprocally.

This is clear enough, but sometimes the two norms conflict and thereby produce a force for change in social customs. For example, how does one address a person who has superior status to oneself, but with whom one is friendly? Similarly, how does one address a person who is of junior status but with whom one feels no bonds of intimacy? Just to take an example of the first problem, how does one address one's boss if he happens to be a close personal friend?

For the most part social awkwardnesses such as this have been worked out by now, although they still crop up from time to time. But some years ago they were more important than at present. Social changes had to occur. Mainly, in the history of social interaction, the solidarity rule has come to surplant the status rule. According to Brown this has probably occurred because society has become more open-class and egalitarian replacing the old feudal society where a man's position was given simply by his birthright.

In general then the status rule has been somewhat suppressed, although it still applies in some situations, where there is a substantial difference in age or occupation for example. Typically, England produced a different solution from the rest of Europe, suppressing one of its pronouns altogether. (Ye was the second person plural – the more distant form – and thou the second person singular – the more familiar. Ye became you and thou disappeared.) Thus in the English language, when there is a social problem due to the conflict of the two rules we can avoid addressing a person by any name at all and the personal pronoun makes no difference.

Social Reflections of Status and Solidarity

In general, balanced symmetrical relationships between people reflect solidarity and imbalanced asymmetrical relationships reflect status, such inequalities being reasonably complex matters. Brown categorises relationships between people into five aspects with respect to status and solidarity. These will be dealt with in turn.

(1) Personal Characteristics

With respect to personal characteristics, status can be dealt with quite
quickly. Any two people can be compared as to their social status. Such
comparisons will depend upon dimensions such as seniority, lineage,
education and income. For the most part, members of society agree
fairly well on one another's social value, even though this is something
which tends to be devalued in modern western society.

Solidarity is more complex than status. Two people are likely to
become solidary (closer, more friendly, etc.) if their personal characteristics are equal (birds of a feather actually do flock together). Also it
has been shown that it is possible to predict the formation of friendship
patterns between people who have never met on the basis of knowledge
about their previous interests, attitudes and values.

These are perhaps fairly obvious points. However, less obvious, until
it is mentioned, is the fact that what has been called a common fate can
lead to immediate increases in solidarity. For example, French moun-
taineers who might not know one another well, switch from using the
mutual '*vous*' form of address to the mutual '*tu*' once they are above
a certain height, and the danger has presumably increased. Think also
of the friendly relationships which are quickly established if you have
ever become stuck in a lift with other people, or stuck between stations
on a train, even if you are waiting with other people to be interviewed
for the same job. Similarly, if people share some fairly extreme physical
characteristic they are likely to rapidly establish a solidarity relationship. Very short or very tall people will get on together quite rapidly,
as also probably will people who share some affliction or illness. The
friendliness which exists between comparative strangers in doctors'
waiting rooms or the casualty department of hospitals is well known.

Occasionally, solidarity can be based on differences rather than
similarities. But the differences will normally be complementary.
This might be seen for example in a relationship between two people
in which one needs to be nurtured and the other enjoys being nurturant.
Or when one person is an invalid and the other does not mind nursing.
By a similar token there are occasions on which similarity does not lead
to increased solidarity. On the face of it, similarity should lead to
increased liking which should lead to more similarity and proximity;
life should get better and better. It does not, because sometimes
similarity leads to very high predictability which in turn can lead to
boredom. Also, from time to time status tends to rear its head. Two
status equals in parallel jobs can be the greatest of friends until their

boss leaves and they are both being considered for his job. Then, either one might be secretly pleased at an increase in his own status at the expense of that of his friend.

(2) Spatial Characteristics

The patterns that people make in space reflect both status and solidarity much as do personal characteristics. With respect to solidarity near and far are symmetrical relations, nearness reflecting friendship and more intimate relationships, and remoteness reflecting social as well as physical distance. Obviously nearness in space is a virtual prerequisite for solidarity as it is necessary to interaction. This is clearly shown by the established fact that nearness of dwelling or unit of work leads to a greater likelihood of friendships developing than does remoteness. As will be mentioned more fully later, friendships most often develop between next door neighbours.

Status is as clearly demonstrated in space as is solidarity. Here the relationship is obviously asymmetrical. If A is above B, then B must be below A; if A is in front of B, then B must be behind A. In many areas of western society above and in front of denote higher status. The person of higher status sits at the head table, or at the head of the table if he lives in a higher part of town. Also he is kept apart from other people in the spaces of his everyday life. So there are VIP lounges at airports, first-class compartments on trains, boxes in theatres, and so on.

It is an easy matter to decide the relationship which exists between two people by observing the patterns they create in space. In general people who know one another well stay physically closer and a person of higher status retains a physically higher position. Spatial relationships are in fact more complex than this, but this matter will be dealt with more fully later in this chapter.

(3) Feelings

The feelings involved in status are self-evident; in one case it is of superiority and in the other inferiority, the former being pleasant and the latter not. Similarly the feelings involved in solidarity are those of joining with someone else, shading into indifference and eventually dislike. As previously, status is asymmetrical and solidarity symmetrical. At least, it has been shown that if A likes B then B will almost certainly like A. However, if A dislikes B then one cannot predict whether or not B will dislike A. Dislike appears not to be symmetrical.

Brown suggests that *sympathy* is often an accompaniment to

solidarity; but to feel sympathy there must be *contact*. It is difficult to feel sympathy and solidarity with the plight of people at the other side of the world. Close and continued contact is necessary. Also, occasional clashes between the feelings involved in status and solidarity can lead to hypocrisy. Take an example used earlier: although we may like and feel sympathy towards a certain friend, we also might be secretly pleased when something happens to depress his status relative to our own.

(4) Behaviour

There have been few studies concerned with the behaviour involved in status and solidarity, perhaps because observations of social behaviour really provided the starting point for discussion of the two dimensions in any case. However, De Soto (1960) carried out one laboratory investigation bearing on the degree to which status and solidarity are asymmetrical and symmetrical behaviourally as well as in other ways.

De Soto had his subjects learn lists of paired associates of the form in which they saw two names on a card and had to anticipate the link between them. For example, two of the names were Bill and Ray and the missing term might be 'confides in', 'does not confide in'. Sometimes the pairs were arranged symmetrically and sometimes not. The symmetrical sets were learned more rapidly than the asymmetrical. This might be because such symmetrical use of the terms themselves might be expected in the English language, or because that is what subjects would expect *behaviourally:* people either confide *mutually* or not at all, they like each other or not at all.

(5) Indirect Expressions

Finally, status and solidarity as dimensions of interpersonal relationships are expressed indirectly by various social symbols which have become customary over the years. For example, solidarity tends to be expressed by similarity in appearance (students with beards, city gentlemen in pin-striped suits, football supporters with matching scarves, etc.) and frequent meetings and conversations. Status is very clearly expressed by possessions; the idea of the status symbol (a bigger car, home, washing-machine, television, etc) has long been known to advertisers and market researchers.

Although such social symbols may seem unnecessary and are easy to denigrate in fact they perform very useful functions. For example, they are important when faced with introduction into a social setting in which we do not know the people. What people tend to do under these conditions is to look around and make a quick evaluation of the relative status and solidarity of the people already in there in order to make interaction with them a smoother matter. For example, it would save social embarrassment if the person who was obviously in charge could be easily picked out by his style of dress or some such indicant. Perhaps the best example is that of a wedding or engagement ring. The sight of such a ring on the hand of someone to whom one is attracted might save · all manner of possible embarrassment.

Finally then, it seems clear that much of our social interaction is governed by rules of status and solidarity, in present times particularly the latter. Although it was illustrated earlier by reference to forms of address, it clearly applies to a very wide range of circumstances. Think of just two simple examples. In Britain, those who know one another well will usually say hello when they meet in the morning, whereas those who are acquaintances will tend to say a mutual good morning. But there are also situations in which one person (the superior) will reply with a 'hallo' to a 'good morning' from his subordinate. Also, there is the matter of social invitations. There is no problem when on the dimension of solidarity, but when it is confused with status, definite patterns emerge, which lead to social awkwardness if broken. It is the superior who must normally bring about the increase in solidarity by issuing the social invitation. If the inferior does so, various social boundaries are torn down.

Social Techniques

Faced with a potential social interaction, most people either consciously or unconsciously abstract whatever information they can in order to make inferences and predictions about the other people involved. Simultaneously the others will be making similar inferences and predictions about them. Such information is gained from two sources: *static* and *dynamic*. Some of the static features of people have been mentioned above and in other chapters. These are characteristics such as body shape, hair length and colour, clothing, and so on. These are relatively unsubtle and uninteresting and do not provide very much detailed or useful or even accurate information. The present section is concerned with dynamic characteristics.

Other than verbal communication, all the behaviours that people engage in socially are basically concerned with communication. They are different kinds of social act, each with its communicative function and each with its own particular features. Recently these acts have been termed *body language*. Fuller discussions of the ideas and research described below may be found in Argyle (1969).

(1) Bodily Contact

The most primitive kind of non-verbal communication involves contact between bodies of two individuals; touching of some sort. It is found in most animals and probably in all but the most unusual of humans. The various meanings which body contact can have are fairly obvious. It can have implications for sexual encounters, aggressive encounters, leading and following.

Almost always body contact means an increase in *intimacy*, an increase in emotional involvement between the interactants, be this pleasant or unpleasant. Most societies have even developed symbolic forms of contact such as hand-shaking, back-slapping, social kissing, and so on. Such symbolic touching tends to occur particularly at the start and finish of social encounters, almost as though the occasion is being marked with an expression of reasonable intimacy and hence friendship between the interactants.

Body contact has been studied descriptively by Jourard (e.g. 1966), his interest centring on who touches whom, where and when; this sort of information being gathered either by close observation or by asking relevant questions. His general findings are fairly self-evident; namely, that there is more touching more often and in more places by those who are in intimate relationships with one another than those who are less intimate. But more interestingly, there are cultural differences in amount of touching, there being more in the Latin and Latin-American countries than in countries such as England. In England the amount of bodily contact between people is at a minimum relative to most other countries which have been studied.

(2) Distance

The distance that people retain between them when they are interacting is mainly important in relation to intimacy and dominance. Hall (1959) made a detailed cross cultural analysis of this and found several interesting relationships. He suggests that people tend to carry around with them a series of physical distances which they regard as appropriate for various types of social interaction. By 'appropriate' is meant those physical distances at which the person feels comfortable during an interaction. If one of these distances is not maintained then the individual will feel edgy socially, be he too near or too far away from the other person.

Of course, appropriate distances also vary with the surroundings. It is perfectly acceptable to stand very close to a stranger in a crowded lift or train, although such distances would not be tolerated between the same two people if they were the only people in a waiting-room. However, to anticipate a later discussion a little, social distance depends on other aspects of non-verbal communication as well. For example, it is acceptable to be very close to a stranger as long as bodily contact is not made and his eyes cannot be seen. So strangers in waiting-rooms will sit quite comfortably back-to-back with only inches separating their heads. Think of the same situation with the two people facing each other.

Again there are large cultural differences in what are regarded as comfortable social distances. Typically, people from the Mediterranean and Latin-American countries stand closer when having a conversation than those from Northern Europe or the USA. So if two such people meet, one is constantly moving closer to achieve his ideal interaction distance, and the other is constantly edging backwards to maintain his ideal distance. A slow dance of this sort can go on throughout an evening, with both interactants no doubt harbouring strange thoughts about each other's motivation.

(3) Gestures

The conscious and unconscious aspects of non-verbal communication are perhaps most easily seen with gestures. Some seem to be overt social techniques which are consciously aimed at communication, and others seem to be made quite involuntarily and may or may not be correctly interpreted by those who see them. Conscious gestures can be quickly dismissed. These are such things as hand movements which are clearly acting as adjuncts to speech, qualifying or modifying it in some way.

Less obvious are characteristics such as body posture which can indicate whether the individual is tense or relaxed. Or bodily orientation by which it is possible to gain an indication of the relationship between two people. For example, competitors tend to face each other whilst those who are co-operating tend to remain at 90 degrees, usually sitting side by side.

As is mentioned in the next chapter it often seems to be the case that emotions which are produced by social interaction and which it is not appropriate to express freely, tend to overflow into involuntary gestures. So a person who is emotionally aroused but having to suppress it may be seen to be biting his nails, rubbing his nose, tugging at his hair or waggling his feet. Most of us have developed such ways of expressing nervous energy and much information can be gleaned about the emotional state of a person by observing when they occur.

(4) Facial Expression and Eye Movements

Facial expression is dealt with at greater length in the next chapter and is mainly concerned with the expression of emotion. It can be reduced to changes in the region of the eyes, the mouth, and the overall shape of the face. Although a person's facial expression appears to be the primary way in which we gauge his emotion, in fact it is quite difficult to be accurate in this without having some knowledge of the situation which led up to it.

However, in the present context, it is *eye movements* which are of more importance. These have an effect on social interaction which is out of all proportion to the amount of effort they require. For example, if A looks at B this means that interaction can proceed. However, if he looks at B for a long glance this can have a variety of meanings, depending on the circumstances; it might be friendly, amorous, aggressive, curious, or so on. In any case, like body contact and increased physical proximity, it clearly indicates a heightening of intimacy of some sort; emotion is involved. This is particularly the case where there is *eye-contact* between people, i.e. when they look into each other's eyes.

One study on this topic involved having a series of two-minute interactions between all the possible pairs of ten people who had previously not met. They were taken and sat down at opposite sides of a table with a screen between them and were instructed that when the screen lifted they were to spend two minutes getting to know each other. Amongst other things it was found that the first thing that happened when the screen lifted was that the two subjects would look into each other's eyes briefly; and the second was that one of them would look away. This was before any conversations began.

It was shown that this breaking of eye-to-eye contact was arranged hierarchically. Thus if B looked away first from eye-to-eye contact with A and if C looked away first from eye-to-eye contact with B, it could be safely predicted that C would look away first from eye-contact with A. Afterwards this was shown to be inversely related to a questionnaire measure of dominance. So he who looked away first was the more likely to be socially dominant. Although this result seems to go against common sense, it takes on meaning when it is realised that people who are talking tend to look away and those who are listening tend to look. Also, he who talks first and talks most in an encounter is likely to be the more dominant. He who looks away from an initial eye encounter is likely to talk first, and so on.

This and very many similar studies have shown that eye-gaze has three major social functions. Clearly, it is expressive of whatever emotion the person is feeling and of increased intimacy. Also however, it serves a *monitoring* function, allowing the individual to make assessments about the other person. And thirdly, it is a *regulator*; by occurring at some times and not at others, eye gaze helps to regulate the course of an interaction. Also, it tends to be in balance with other aspects of non-verbal communication, at least according to Argyle. There seems to be an amount of touching, physical proximity and eye-to-eye contact with which each individual is comfortable in each social setting. When one of these over- or under-shoots then he will tend to compensate by decreasing or increasing one of the others. For example, if a person is touched more than he finds comfortable socially, then he will tend to avert his gaze more than he would normally.

(5) Indirect Aspects of Speech

Apart from its obvious communicational intent, speech, in its non-linguistic aspects provides one of the most subtle examples of the unintentional information that people give one another. For example, the *patterns* of speech and silence vary between people enormously, and individuals develop their own characteristic ways of responding to interruption or silence. For example, some people raise their voices and talk down an interruption whereas others yield at once when interrupted. Some people seem to be quite comfortable with long silences in a conversation; others will fill any silence with anything, no matter how trivial.

Also, of course, the same words can be said in quite different ways to carry vastly different meanings. We make everyday judgements of such differences constantly, usually of the person's emotional state. At the extreme, most people have probably had the experiences of hearing a 'no' said in a way such that it actually means 'yes', and a 'yes' put such that it unmistakably means 'no'.

Social Styles

The five aspects of social behaviour described in the last section can be seen simply as that: types of social act. Or they can be seen as social techniques which are sometimes used in an overtly manipulative manner to gain a person whatever he might desire socially. Probably for any individual these three alternatives are appropriate descriptions at different times and occasions in his social life. Be this as it may, the various elements tend to be gathered together in any one person into a general style of social responding. Although of course, each one of us is unique socially, many social styles can be roughly categorised into two main types — the affiliative and the dominant.

(1) The Affiliative Style

The affiliative style involves close physical proximity, increased bodily contact, a great deal of eye contact and smiling, a friendly tone of voice, and conversation which centres on personal topics. From this brief description it should be clear to make a conscious attempt to develop this style requires a great deal of subtlety. If any of the elements were taken too far, all but the most timorous of people would back out of the situation as fast as they could. Intimate, affiliative relationships only develop if both parties can obtain some rewards from the interaction.

(2) The Dominant Style

Sometimes the dominant style is used as a seemingly natural part of a person's social repertoire; other people (such as some in public life for example) use it professionally, and yet others cannot seem to avoid being dominated. It involves speaking loudly, fast and for most of the time; interrupting others and taking every opportunity to influence rather than be influenced. When having to listen rather than talk, an attentive unsmiling facial expression is adopted. Again, if all this is turned on at once only the most submissive of people would not extricate themselves from the situation. So, to establish a truly dominant relationship, more subtlety is required, and the behaviours mentioned have to be mixed up with those involved in increasing affiliation. The other person must be given some incentive to stay.

The descriptions above have been put as though the individual involved is consciously attempting to develop a particular style of social behaviour. No doubt this does occur from time to time. But usually such styles develop as an integral part of the person's upbringing, and are not thought about at all consciously. Whatever social skills and techniques or social behaviours are employed, they are all highly dependent on feedback from the other people with whom the person comes into contact.

Other than to say that social skills are learned (see Chapter 14) there is little else that can be said about the source of an individual's particular social style. Certainly, it is related to personality (extroverts have typically different patterns of social interaction than introverts for example), but this does not get us very far. Also, social behaviour changes with age, showing gradual improvement. And in general women tend to be more affiliative and dependent than men who tend to be more aggressive and dominant than women.

Interpersonal Relationships as a Social Skill

One of Argyle's main theoretical contributions to an understanding of social interaction is his idea that it can be looked at as very much akin to a motor skill such as driving a car or typing. His argument is that much of social behaviour is like that involved in motor behaviour, but that it has a few qualities which set it apart from this as well.

Similarities Between Social and Motor Skills

(1) Aims. Both social and motor skills have definite aims. For example the aim of a driver is to direct a car along the road safely, or to get from London to Manchester. In a very similar way a person engaging in social skills has definite aims, which are linked to his motivations and rewards just as they would be in motor skills. For example the aim of teaching is to convey knowledge, of interviewing to obtain information, of salesmanship to change attitudes, of rearing a child to change personality, of nursing to supervise and nurture, of therapy to change behaviour, and so on. Similarly, in everyday life, a person interacting has certain aims about the interaction, to develop a friendly or a dominant relationship for example.

(2) Perception. In the pursuit of a motor skill perception has to be selective; the person has to learn what to attend to and has to become sensitive to these cues. So a person playing tennis has to learn to attend to the flight, speed and direction of the ball, his opponent's position on court, and the movements of his opponent's arm and body. It is no use watching the net or looking at the tramlines. In motor skills there is a vast amount of selecting, organising and interpreting of incoming information.

Similar processes are important in social skills. If the aim is to establish a new relationship with a member of the opposite sex there is little profit in attending to someone else, or the weather, or your own cigarette smoking. Attention should be paid to the other person and what he or she is saying, and the intricate non-verbal information he or she is providing. Again, in this context it is the eyes and the direction and length of their gaze which will be of prime importance.

(3) Organisation. In both motor and social skills any information which is gathered in has to be organised centrally. There must therefore be a

store of rules (either verbalised or unverbalised) in the brain which will allow some sort of translation to occur. So, in driving one learns what to do in order to cope with various road conditions, such as fog or snow. Similarly in social skills one learns how to cope with different types of input. For example one learns how to deal with a person who says very little: by asking open-ended questions, talking of what interests him, and being very encouraging of anything he does say, for instance.

(4) Motor responses. In motor skills eventually the brain sends out messages to the muscles and behaviour results. So it is with social skills. People have to learn to control their tone of voice, their gestures, and in fact their general style of social behaviour.

(5) Feedback. An essential part of motor skills is their continual modification on the basis of feedback. A driver knows when he has done something wrong and corrects; similarly a tennis player knows he has made a poor stroke when he sees the ball fly out of court. He learns from this and plays the stroke differently on the next occasion.

So it is with social skills. We continuously monitor our own performances socially and change them or not as appropriate. If you realise that you are pleasing someone or displeasing someone then you carry on in the same way in the one case and cease in the other. Feedback is important socially although it is sometimes more difficult to come by than it is in motor skills.

(6) Timing. Finally, motor and social skills are alike in that they both depend very much on timing and rhythm. To continue with the previous examples, in driving or playing tennis it is important to have precise anticipation of when and how to make a particular response. The same is true of social interaction. People must learn to speak in turn rather than together, they must learn how much and when it is appropriate to touch another person in their culture, and so on. They must in fact learn to share interaction time according to the rules and conventions of the culture in which they live.

Social Skills – Unique Features

The features of social skills which set them apart from motor skills exist for the obvious reason that social skills involve more than one person; they depend on interaction between people rather than on interaction between man and machine or man and apparatus.

(1) Rapport. The exercise of social skill always involves the need to establish rapport with the other person; to develop a sensitive, understanding relationship. Argyle argues that there are three aspects to this: (a) a clear channel of communication between the interactants, (b) a degree of mutual trust and acceptance, and (c) a smooth pattern of interaction.

Whatever he might be attempting to do an operator of social skills will not achieve it unless he can establish *rapport*. This is so whether he is trying to persuade his child that one course of action is better than another or he is selling insurance from door to door. Clearly, rapport is not an all or none affair, it requires different degrees for different situations. You need more *rapport* with someone to ask them about their sexual life than you do to ask them if you can borrow a comb.

Those who are concerned with training others in social skills for their jobs agree that the following are important in establishing rapport: (a) a friendly manner, (b) cutting down social barriers, (c) establishing smooth interaction patterns, (d) finding areas of common interest, (e) showing a sympathetic interest, and (f) meeting the other person on his own ground, that is using his words for things and his manner of expression.

(2) Consideration. Other than routine servicing and maintenance, a car driver does not have to consider the state of his vehicle. However a person exercising social skills has to find ways of keeping the other person involved. If the other person does not like what is happening he can just withdraw. Again Argyle argues that three techniques seem to produce the right effect. (a) If A cannot do all that B wants then he must find some other means of rewarding him. (b) Smiling and nodding for appropriate behaviour are effective reinforcers, as also is gentle persuasion rather than direct orders. (c) A should resist B's influence.

(3) Motivation. A driver does not have to motivate his car or a tennis player his racket. On the other hand a person exercising social skills often has to motivate the other person. If for example he wants someone to buy something or to fill in a questionnaire, or to come out to a dance with him, he has to arouse the appropriate motivation. By a similar token he has to try to alleviate any anxiety the other person may be experiencing.

(4) Impressions. A driver or a tennis player does not set out to impress his car or racket. This provides a very clear contrast with social skills

in which the performer is often much concerned with the impression he is making.

Whether Argyle's idea of drawing a parallel between motor skills and social skills is useful remains to be seen. Motor skills certainly provide a reasonable analogue as far as they go. On the other hand it should be clear from the above that the analogy is by no means complete. Also it may be that there are differences between the use of social skills in a professional sense, i.e as part of the individual's job, and their rather more haphazard use in everyday life. Certainly the everyday life situation is often much less contrived and less well thought out. Nevertheless it may be that similar princples are involved. Discussion of the way in which social skills are learned and taught will be reserved for a later chapter.

Summary Points

(1) Interpersonal relationships depend on communication and appear to be governed by certain rules which are understood at least implicitly within a particular culture.

(2) Two important aspects of social encounters are status (involving dominance) and solidarity (or intimacy). The way in which norms for these facets of interaction are reflected can be simply expressed in the way in which people address one another when they interact. Nowadays, solidarity seems to be more important as a governor of social relationships than does status.

(3) Both status and solidarity are reflected in personal characteristics, spatial characteristics, feelings, behaviour and social symbols.

(4) Interpersonal relationships can be seen as a matter of the development and use of social techniques, either knowingly or unknowingly. Often these amount to questions of non-verbal aspects of communication.

(5) Non-verbal communication involves touching, spatial position, body posture and gesture, facial expression and direction of eye gaze, and the various non-verbal aspects of speech. In general an increase in any of these facets of communication means an increase in intimacy, be this shaded in the direction of sex or aggression or friendship. Also, the various behaviours seem to be in a sort of balance.

(6) The various subtleties of non-verbal communication tend to be gathered together for the individual into his own style of interaction. The two most common of these are the affiliative and the dominant style.

(7) Argyle argues that social interaction and interpersonal relationships

can be viewed as involving social skills which in many of their defining characteristics are similar to motor skills. However, in spite of these similarities, social skills have certain aspects of their own, largely because unlike motor skills they directly involve other people.

Study Questions – 12

(1) Is it possible for a patient to be with a member of one of the caring professions and not communicate with her (him)? What are the implications of your answer for your professional role?

(2) Think of patients with whom you have worked and describe their particular styles of non-verbal communication. What examples can you find of what look like overflows of nervous energy into aimless movement?

(3) Make some observations of interactions between yourself (and your colleagues) and your patients. Having done this and recorded what you see, attempt to alter the course of conversations by smiling more or less often or by looking at the other person's eyes more or less often. Can you move a person around a room (without his knowledge) by infringing his personal space?

(4) How generally important in your job do you think the subtleties of social behaviour to be? Does your job involve the employment of social skills? How?

(5) Does the interpersonal behaviour of people change when they are hospitalised or in some way incapacitated? Does the interpersonal behaviour of people change when they *work* in institutional settings?

(6) From your knowledge of previous interactions with patients and colleagues, which do you believe to be the more important for communication, verbal or non-verbal behaviour? Do they communicate different things or the same things in different ways? What implications do your answers have for your professional role?

(7) When dealing with patients have you ever noticed that some of them will not look you in the eye? What reasons do you think they would have for this, and do you think that they would be aware of it?

(8) Do you think that the reading of the type of material to be found in this chapter will bring about changes in your own social behaviour? If so, is this a good thing for your professional role, or not?

(9) Try to analyse some social situations with patients and colleagues in which you have been embarrassed or have come away feeling guilty. What went wrong? Why? How was it reflected non-verbally?

(10) How important to your relationship with a patient do you think

your initial encounter is? What might you do about this encounter in order to set the scene so that you could be maximally effective in your professional role?

13 JUDGEMENTS AND IMPRESSIONS OF PERSONALITY

As was seen earlier, perception can be viewed as having two major aspects: being selective and recoding any data into a memorisable form, and then using this information as a basis on which to make predictions, this in turn helping to minimise surprise. Thus it is with the process of forming impressions of personality and character; there is movement from making observations of behaviour and physical characteristics to making inferences about personality.

Any judgements that we make about other people are all made as inferences from what they look like and what they do. Often such judgements are unconscious and based on the person's clothes, hair, build, and then on more dynamic features such as the various aspects of non-verbal communication described previously, particularly facial expression. It is this that we use to make judgements about emotion and hence of personality.

Before going on to describe some of the research and ideas concerning impression formation it is important to point out one methodical difficulty. To study some people making judgements of others in a laboratory is clearly very artificial. Usually they have to write down their judgements, either by checking off words from a list, or by choosing the appropriate trait from pairs of opposites, or even by writing a free description. All of this following some stimulus which can vary anywhere from the sound of someone's voice or a line drawing of a human figure to actual confrontation with a person.

There is always the problem of whether or not such techniques of study allow an understanding of the process of impression formation as it goes on in everyday life. All that can be said is that such laboratory tasks simulate the real-life situation. In both the laboratory and the outside world inferences are made from present behaviour and appearance and these are used to work out probabilities of future behaviour and hence expectancies about personality and character. In either situation if expectancies are not borne out then people tend to be surprised. The problem of methodology will be returned to later when discussing the question of whether or not some people are more accurate than others in their judgements of personality. It is in this important area that investigation is most difficult.

First Impressions

An appropriate starting point for a discussion of how people form impressions of one another's personality is with the question of first impressions; are these of fundamental importance? do they override later impressions? are our parents right to point out the dangers of first impressions? as parents no doubt have for generations.

It is sufficient to describe the work of one man on first impressions, since it sets the scene so well. Luchins (1957) composed a passage of descriptive prose in which a person had to face a number of decisions and could take various courses of action following these decisions. He composed the passage so that it could be simply rewritten such that in one case the person behaved as a typical extrovert and in the other as a typical introvert. He then gave these two passages to different groups of subjects and asked them to write personality profiles about the hypothetical person and to answer specific questions about his personality. The impressions created by the two passages were vastly different, as Luchins had wanted.

Now, the way in which the passages had been written was such that they could be put together as one long passage, and this could be done in either order; the extrovert or the introvert passage could come first and either way perfectly good sense would be made. Luchins put together the two passages in this way and gave them to more subjects for their judgements of personality. The question he was asking was: which would be more important in their judgements, *primacy* (first impressions) or *recency* (later impressions)?

Luchins' general finding was that primacy was the more important; it was the first impressions gained (from the first halves of the joined passages) which had the important effect. This being so there would obviously be some discrepancies between the impressions the subjects formed and the latter halves of the descriptions. When Luchins faced the subjects with these discrepancies they would justify their judgements by saying things like: earlier on, the hypothetical individual was 'acting in character' and for some reason out of character later on. Or something unpleasant must have happened to him, which was not described, in order to bring about the later, uncharacteristic behaviour.

At this point then it seemed that the first impressions have a fairly extreme effect. However, Luchins found that such effects could be overcome quite easily. This could be done in two ways. Either by warning subjects beforehand of the danger of first impressions, or by putting in some extra activity between their reading of the two halves of the joined passages. As these are more like the situation which obtains in real life — people do warn one another of the dangers of first impressions and do all manner of other things between their inter-actions with particular people — it may be that recency is more important than primacy.

Although Luchins created an ingenious investigation into first impressions, what he cannot tell us is whether or not first impressions are likely to be more or less accurate than later impressions. As will be seen later it is virtually impossible to answer this question, even though in everyday life, for many reasons, it is usually assumed that first impressions are less accurate than later ones.

Centrality

As well as the order in which impressions are formed, there are many sources of influence on the matter of how we make our perceptions of other people, including of course our own personalities. As an example of such sources of influence, there is the likelihood that some traits appear to be more important than others in judgements. If a person is judged to have a particular characteristic then this will make it very likely that he will be judged to have other characteristics as well. Such traits are said to be central.

Work on centrality began with a long series of investigations by Asch (1946). These took the form of reading to his subjects lists of traits which were supposed to apply to an individual. For example in one case the traits were: intelligent, skilful, industrious, warm, determined, practical, cautious. On the basis of these traits subjects were asked to give a brief description of the person. For some subjects the word 'warm' in the list was replaced with the word 'cold'. Subjects also had to pick which of a number of pairs of opposite characteristics applied to the person.

Asch's general finding was that the presence of 'warm' or 'cold' in the original list made a vast difference to the judgements made by his subjects; far more difference in fact than if he replaced any of the other traits by their opposites, intelligent/unintelligent, skilful/clumsy for example. Asch therefore described warm/cold as *central* traits, central because they were so strongly important to impressions derived from the list. He also gained evidence for the centrality of other pairs of traits such as polite/blunt.

The importance of 'warm' was even seen when it was embedded in a list of very negative words (vain, shrewd, unscrupulous, shallow, envious). Presented with this, subjects seemed to distinguish two levels of reality. They assumed that the person *appeared* to be warm rather

than being actually warm. As well as making very good sense from
everyday experience, this also points to the importance of warm and
cold as determinants of the judgements made of others. If for example
'unscrupulous' had been replaced by 'scrupulous' subjects would not
have had the same necessity to distinguish between reality and appearances.

Emotional Expression and Recognition

Having introduced the subject of impressions of personality by discussing first impressions and centrality, we come to what is the single
most important aspect of the subject; how people express emotion and
recognise such expressions in one another. This has a central position
for a number of reasons: (1) emotional expression contains a great deal
of useful information, (2) emotional expression changes constantly and
yet can be suppressed, (3) everyone can recognise emotional expressions
in others, but how? since emotion is such a very private experience.

In the discussion which follows mention will not be made of the
work of very many specific psychologists. The reason for this is that
there has been a great deal of work in this area and the list of names
would become rather unwieldy. The work is summarised in detail in
Frijda (1969), Izard (1972) or Strongman (1978). Apart from its
obvious importance, another reason why there has been a great deal of
work on emotional expression is the difficulty there is in studying it at
all; it presents a challenge. As was mentioned in the chapter on emotion,
it is very difficult to reproduce 'real' emotion in an artificial laboratory
situation. Nowhere is this more evident than in research on emotional
expression.

There have been very many creative attempts to overcome the artificiality problem, often involving skilled actors or draughtsmen or
electronic equipment. However, much of the scene setting was achieved
many years ago in a very early study. It will help to describe this briefly.
The investigator made films of twelve people whilst they were either
acting their responses to or giving genuine responses to stimuli such as:
hearing the blast of a horn, having an electric shock, treading on a snail,
hearing a joke, and so on. The films were given to subjects in order that
they match them to a list of the situations.

In general the findings were that accuracy depended on who was
making the judgement, how much of the face on the film he was per-
mitted to see, and whether the expression was natural or acted. It
appeared that empathy was the main route to judgement; subjects tried
to place themselves as the person in the film and to imagine how they

would have responded to the various situations. However, for the moment the main point is that this study exemplifies the sort of manner in which the artificiality problem has been overcome.

Dimensions of Expression

One of the most influential ways in which the attempt has been made to understand the judgement of emotional expression has involved the idea of dimensions of emotion. One suggestion was that all emotional expression and recognition could be represented with just three dimensions:

(1) pleasantness/unpleasantness
(2) attention/rejection
(3) level of activation (from sleep to high arousal)

The idea is that these three dimensions underlie any emotional expression and are therefore the basis of any judgements we make of such expressions. If for example one thinks of the expression of anger it could be characterised as unpleasant, rejecting and involving high tension. The expression of happiness on the other hand would be pleasant, attentive and aroused.

Although the idea of dimensions of expression and recognition has the appeal of parsimony about it, the problem has been that different investigators have 'discovered' different numbers of dimensions. So for example very often researchers have found no good evidence for the attention/rejection dimension, and others have found up to six dimensions.

The basic problem here is that we cannot distinguish the various emotions from one another by their expressions as precisely as we can with words, and even with words it is often very difficult. Confusion arises because different emotions can lead to very similar expressions (disgust and contempt for example) and different expressions can result from one emotion (think for example of the different ways of registering happiness). On top of this each individual tends to have his own idiosyncratic ways of expressing particular emotions. It is even difficult to say under what conditions emotions are expressed clearly (and hence recognised more easily) and when they are not.

Movement

As is no doubt apparent by now, very often emotional expression and its judgement is studied using photographs of fixed expressions. This is perhaps one of the greatest artificialities since in real life judgements are made in dynamic situations of constant change. One of the important aspects of judging emotions might therefore be movement.

A start was made in the study of this area in the 1950s, reducing investigations to a very simple level. An observer is shown a piece of apparatus in which there is a horizontal slot through which he can see two small coloured rectangles. These can be moved along the slot with speed, direction and extent of movement under the control of the experimenter. The result is very similar to watching a cartoon film in which there are only coloured moving lights and shapes. The observer tends to give the shapes a personification and to imbue them with emotional significance, see them as having a purpose, and so on.

For example, if one rectangle moves slowly along the slot until it touches the other and the second then moves to and fro for a moment and then moves rapidly away, then an observer will tend to see the second rectangle running from the first in fear. Frequently subjects in such studies make their judgements by referring to the emotional state of the rectangles. The implication seems to be that when emotional expression is characterised as simply as this it can be easily separated into its *positive* (approach, and contact) and *negative* (escape, withdrawal, avoidance) aspects. As might be expected speed is also important; fast movement indicates violence and slow movement tranquillity and calm.

Although these studies have not been taken very far and have their obvious limitations, they do show the importance of movement in emotional expression and recognition. In fact it is easy to see this in everyday life, if attention is paid to the manner in which people move when they are interacting. All becomes clear if one sees a film of movement speeded up, with changes of direction and speed compressed more in time than they usually would be. Patterns of approach and withdrawal become obvious. Of course, it would be wrong to suggest that the complexities of emotional expression could be reduced to this rather elemental level. However it is true to say that movement is an important part of the recognition of expressions.

Context

In everyday life any expression of emotion occurs within a particular social context. We usually make our judgements of an expression in the knowledge of what led up to the expression, where it is occurring, and with previous experience of the person doing the expressing. It is likely that these are all cues that help in making judgements. For example, the knowledge that a person was going to have a major operation on the following day would allow his emotional expressions to be interpreted more easily. Similarly if a stranger came running round the corner, his face very white and strained, you would interpret his expressions very differently if he was followed by a gang of youths than if he were chasing someone who had stolen his wallet.

The context of emotion is important in allowing us to make a check on our judgements of it. There seem to be two processes at work. An initial judgement is made of the expression alone and then we check this a little more precisely against the context in which it occurs. He looks frightened. Is that correct? Should he be frightened? What has made him frightened? If these questions get reasonable answers (reasonable that is in terms of our own experiences) then our initial judgement is endorsed. If for example a mother hears her child suddenly scream out she can probably judge from the sound whether the child is hurt or on the other hand merely angry or frustrated. Then she will have a quick look at the situation he is in, to check her judgement so that she can do whatever is appropriate.

At one time it was thought that context was all important and that judgements of emotional expression could not be made without it. However, this is not so as has been established by studies in which the context and the expression have been set up against each other. People are capable of making judgements of expression when they cannot see the context, although they are not quite as accurate under these conditions. However, one can ask which of the two is the more important in the making of judgements. If one man threatens another with a knife and the threatened man smiles happily, what do we believe?

This situation has been studied by showing people films in which emotions are being expressed and dubbing various (incorrect) sound-tracks onto the films. When this occurs people believe the behaviour rather than the context. They seem to be quick to modify their interpretations of the context to fit the judgement of the person or his expression. Perhaps this is not surprising since the essence of emotional expression must be behaviour. Going back to the previous example, the observer might well say that the person being attacked with a knife knows something that he (the observer) does not, and that is why he is smiling gently. He might for example know that he is so competent at unarmed combat that he will get the knife from the other man with no danger to himself and is welcoming the opportunity to make the attempt.

It is perhaps surprising in some ways that expression should so much dominate context. There are after all four possible ways in which discrepancies between the two could be reduced. One could: (1) divorce the emotion from the situation, (2) divorce the emotion from the situation and simply accept the situation, (3) divorce the expression from the emotion and (4) as most people seem to do, deny the (apparent) situation.

Deception

There are many occasions in everybody's life when it seems best not to display true feelings or not to display feelings at all. These are attempts at outright deception, even though they might occur so automatically in some contexts and to be virtually unconscious. How do people achieve this deception in their expressions? Are some people more successful than others? How do they give themselves away?

Ekman and Friesen (1969) have produced some very interesting ideas on these problems. Basically, their suggestion is that although we make serious attempts to control emotions, these *leak out* in ways of which we might not be aware and which the keen observer can pick up.

It is *gesture* and general *bodily movement* that are important in the context of emotional deception. However, before describing this it is important to say that emotional deceptions can become extremely complex. Think for example of an ongoing interaction between two members of a family in which each is attempting to deceive the other about his true feelings. However each knows what the other is trying to do, and each knows that the other knows. This results in an extraordinarily complicated interaction in which it becomes very difficult to sort out the various levels. The situation becomes further complicated through individual differences in emotional expression and particularly in the ability to conceal it. Some people (even in our culture) express emotion quite openly and others rarely move a muscle.

Ekman and Friesen's basic argument is that the various areas of our bodies have different potentialities for sending non-verbal signals, the face being the best, the hands and arms next, and the feet and legs the worst. We pay attention to these areas accordingly. If a friend has an enraged facial expression you might well ask him why. On the other hand if he kept jogging his leg up and down under the table, even if you were to notice it, you might be a little reticent to comment. Unwittingly we seem to realise these differences between the various areas of the body and to pay attention to them accordingly when trying to conceal emotional expression. Many people become quite adept at controlling the facial expression of emotion, but it is their hands and feet which give them the lie. We pay less attention to the control of our hand and feet movements and it is therefore through these that our emotional state leaks. The judicious observer can tell a great deal from watching the hand and feet movements of what appears to be an otherwise calm person.

Cultural Differences

The question of whether emotional expressions are similar from one culture to the next is actually an attempt to answer a much more basic question. That is, are the expressions of emotion innate, or are they acquired early in life? If there is little variation in emotion between the cultures then it is probably that emotional expression is determined largely innately. The evidence on this question points both ways. Some studies have pointed to cultural differences in emotional expression and others have pointed to similarities. However, it would seem that in general there are marked similarities in the major emotional expressions which are seen throughout the world.

Differences do exist from one culture to the next in the extent to which emotions are openly expressed or are concealed, at least in public. This was demonstrated in a study in which an emotion-evoking film was shown to Japanese and Americans. When members of these cultures watched the film whilst they were alone, there were very little differences in their emotional expressions. However, when they watched the film in company, the Americans expressed their emotions as they had done while alone, whereas the Japanese inhibited their facial expressions quite severely. It is not then that there is any basic difference in the means of emotional expression between these two cultures, but merely in the extent to which their members will openly give vent to the expressions.

Perhaps the most interesting line of evidence on universality in emotional expression comes from studies of blind people. The general finding is that blind and sighted people express emotion very similarly although the blind have a slightly more limited *range* of expression than the sighted. This must be evidence for an important innate component in emotional expression; if emotional expression were learned it would have to be through observation. Interestingly, in passing it is worth noting that contrary to popular belief the blind are *not* better than the sighted at making judgements of emotion from such cues as tone of voice. Certainly they pay more attention to these aspects of things, but they are not better at it.

It should be clear from this discussion that emotional expression and its recognition is an integral part of making judgements about other people. There seems to exist some immediate interpretation of expressive meaning. Recognition occurs very quickly although knowledge and experience are important to it. The whole process depends on cues which come from the obvious facial expression, the less obvious movements of the remainder of the body (cues of non-verbal communication in general) and the even less obvious static features of the individual.

Accuracy

This extended discussion of emotional expression and recognition leads onto some very basic questions in this general area of person perception. How accurate are people when they make judgements of others, be these judgements of their emotional expressions or not? Are some people more accurate than others, and if so why? In some of the studies of emotional expression accuracy was easy enough to assess. If an actor has posed an emotion for a photograph, then what he has posed is the emotion and any discrepancy between this and the subject's judgement reflects inaccuracy. In other studies it is not so simple. One needs to know what an individual's personality is 'really' before being able to say whether a judge's evaluation of it is accurate or not. And as mentioned in the chapter on personality, at present this is impossible.

Leaving aside for the moment the difficulties involved in studying accuracy in the perception of others, Brown (1966) puts forward three reasons why one person might *seem* to be more accurate than the next.

(1) Projection. It is a very common tendency to assume that other people are like ourselves, and to use one's knowledge of oneself as a basis for judging others. Therefore of two people who are making judgement one might seem to be more accurate than the other simply because he was more similar to the person they were both judging. For example, most people *by definition* fall within an average range on personality traits. If a person is himself average then he might judge others as being so, and on simple statistical grounds he might well be right.

(2) Knowledge of a Group. Any one judge may appear to be more accurate than another because he has a good knowledge of the *average* position of the group to which the person being judged belongs. Thus a lecturer might very well be more accurate when judging a student's personality than would someone from outside the educational establishment. This has been shown to be the case when the person with the extra knowledge does not even see the person he is judging.

(3) Response Sets. An individual might have a particular way of judging

people which in certain instances is so appropriate that it makes him seem more accurate than he would normally be. For example, a person who tends to be somewhat conservative in his judgements is more likely to seem accurate than one who is more variable. This again is simply because most people fall somewhere in the average position with respect to most traits.

It is worth bearing in mind these three possibilities in any consideration of accuracy. Even when evidence is established in support of accuracy, it still *might* be spurious. Nevertheless there have been two main questions asked about accuracy. Is accuracy a general skill? What are the qualities of a good judge of personality and character?

These questions, although important, cannot be answered at all definitively. Firstly, the evidence about accuracy as a general skill points in both directions. It can be best summarised by saying that *stereotype* accuracy (predicting for people in general) does seem to be a general skill, whereas *differential* accuracy does not (that is predicting for individuals).

Even more confused is the answer to the second question. The generality of accuracy must have logical priority over the qualities of a good judge. If generality is not established what sense does it make to ask what makes a good judge? One would not even know if good judges exist. However, this logical difficulty has not stopped research being carried out. Such as there is, points to good judges of personality having only two qualitites which show themselves across various studies. (1) Similarity between themselves and those whom they are judging, and (2) self-insight (as rated by others). Both of these characteristics might give the spurious impression of accuracy as described above. As yet then it is impossible to say if some people are better judges of personality than others (although everyday experience suggests that they are) or to say what makes a good judge.

Interpersonal Attraction

One of the most important aspects of person perception and the judgement of others is concerned with interpersonal attraction. What makes two people become attracted to each other? This is a very far-reaching question extending as it does from the making of small talk (why prefer to do this with one person than another?) to romantic love at the other extreme. The obvious and simple answer here is that such interactions are rewarding and this leads to increased attraction which leads to more association and interactions which leads to more attraction, and so small-talk ends up with romantic love. But of course it is not as simple as this since things go wrong, and fortunately not all small talk ends in romantic love. There have been a number of different explanations suggested for interpersonal attraction. The more important of these will be dealt with in turn. (See Secord and Backman 1974, and Berscheid and Walster, 1969 for more extended discussions.)

Persons

One major type of explanation of attraction has dwelt on *similarity* between individuals, although there have been three separate accounts given of this.

(1) Balance. Balance theory is represented in diagram 13.1 in which A and B represent persons, X is some object (such as an interest or an attitude or a belief) and the arrowed lines represent positive and negative reactions. The major argument is that any imbalance in the situation will produce a force to recreate a balance and thus lead to one of the changes characterised in the diagrams. In general, the greater the importance of the object (X), the greater the potential attraction between the two people.

Figure 13.1: Balance Theory

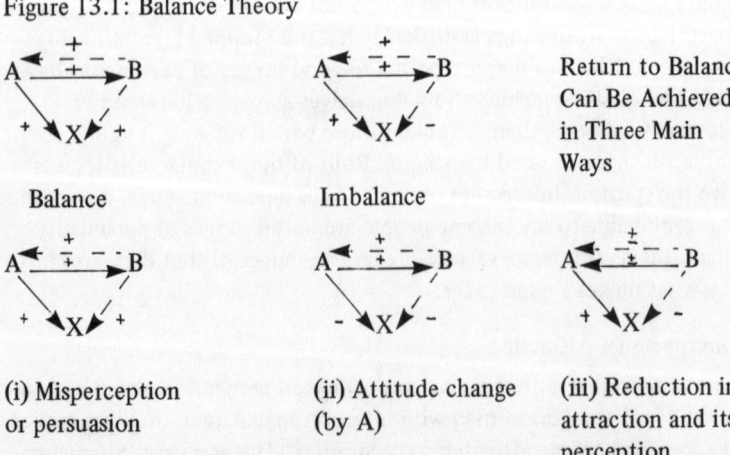

Balance   Imbalance

Return to Balance Can Be Achieved in Three Main Ways

(i) Misperception or persuasion   (ii) Attitude change (by A)   (iii) Reduction in attraction and its perception

Balance theory (deriving from Newcombe. 1961) predicts that there will be a fast and strong attraction between people if they share similar attitudes. Also, if A likes B, then he will predict that B likes him; especially if he judges B as seeing him (A) as he sees himself. The problem with balance theory is that it is difficult to make precise predictions from it; it explains *too* much. It might well be important in situations in which social/emotional needs predominate (see Chapter 16 on leadership and groups) but will be less important when the task is of prime concern.

(2) Reinforcement. Byrne and Nelson (1965) gave subjects an attitude scale and then had them make judgements of other people on the basis of limited information. This information purportedly came from another attitude scale that the person being judged had supposedly completed. Of course, this information was constructed by the experimenters with their knowledge of the attitudes of those who were to make the judgements.

They found that attraction was very dependent (in a directly proportional way) with the number of items on the attitude scale that those doing the judging thought that they had in common with those whom they were judging. Although this result was supported in a number of ways, it may be because the other individual's attitudes are valued by the judge rather than because they are perceived as being similar to them.

(3) Anticipation. If I perceive you to have similar attitudes to mine then this might well make me believe that you would like me, and through this to like you. There is strong empirical support for this view of the anticipation of being liked leading to immediate liking.

Needs

Winch (1958) in a study of how people select mates puts forward the argument that those with complementary needs are attracted. He suggests two reasons for this. (1) Those with complementary needs manage to achieve some gratification of both sets of needs. For example, the person with a great desire to mother and the person with a great desire to be mothered both gain from an association. (2) Each person is attracted to the other because the other fulfils some ideal picture he has of what it would be best to be like.

As might be expected the evidence for this view is fairly weak. It certainly leaves out some considerations. For example there are many instances of people with very similar needs being attracted. Also one's apparent needs might well change according to the social circumstances and the role that one is playing within them.

Interaction

(1) Validation. Secord and Backman best argue this view of attraction themselves. The suggestion is that if we perceive another person as being similar to ourselves then this satisfies a drive to make correct assessments of social reality, which in turn leads to increased liking. I am a person with certain characteristics; if he is like me I must be a properly viable person, and since he has allowed me to make that judgement, I like him.

The point here then is that people are most attracted to those who allow them to maintain a congruent picture of the social world. This can occur in two ways. (a) By *implication*; if he behaves like me then this is confirming that my behaviour is acceptable and good, (b) by *validation*; his behaviour leads me to behave in ways which make me seem good and true.

(2) Dissonance. The theory of cognitive dissonance will be explored in some detail in the next chapter in the section on attitude change. For now, briefly it can be argued that if two things are dissonant and one of these is whether one likes or dislikes another person, the dissonance can be reduced by changing one's likes and dislikes. That it is important to change dissonance, but that the theory cannot predict exactly how the change would be brought about is presented in the next chapter.

(3) Reinforcement. Reinforcement theory of attraction is very straight-forward. The suggestion is that if person A receives rewards in the presence of person B, he will react to these. Any response he so makes will become conditioned to whatever discriminative stimuli are in the environment at the time, including the actual person (B). B will eventually evoke such responses merely by his presence. And the same will be so for B in the presence of A, thus allowing the development of mutual attraction. By a similar analysis of punishment it would be possible to account for lack of attraction or the cooling off of a relationship.

Exchange Theory

Exchange theory will be mentioned in the next chapter since it bears on social learning as well as on interpersonal attraction. It concentrates on relationships between individuals and defines attraction as a function of the *degree to which interactions lead those involved to gain a reward/cost balance which is above some minimum.* So attraction will follow when the rewards which come from the interaction outweigh the costs by some specific amount.

In this context a reward is any activity of one person that gratifies another person's needs. Costs on the other hand include punishments, deterrents in interaction such as fatigue, anxiety, embarrassment, and so on. The reward/cost level must be above some point which the person feels to be his due for some reason — a comparison level. Only then will attraction result. The comparison level is determined by previous experiences of a similar nature, perceptions of what the other interactants are gaining from the situation and a perception of the reward/cost balance in other social situations.

Exchange theory has much to say in some detail about many levels of mutual attraction, and in this perhaps goes further than the other theories.

(1) If two people have similar social backgrounds and values, this establishes high rewards at low cost. Such it is with similarities in abilities and personality traits as well. Also, the greater the opportunity to interact, the lower is the cost of interaction.

(2) In the beginnings of a *friendship* a person might sample the inter-actions and estimate the reward/cost outcomes. He then commits himself to those with the highest outcome. If one considers that both people are doing this then it becomes something of a bargaining match with reward being exchanged for reward, and cost balancing where necessary. Eventually of course as the relationship develops all these processes become institutionalised.

(3) In *intense* relationships such as those of romantic love, the rewards eventually become exclusive. There appear to be some conditions which lead people to be highly susceptible to romantic love. These will include for example: a low comparison level for needing emotional support, which might come for example from general insecurity, a broken love affair, a gradual decline in social rewards, and so on.

Of course relationships change and exchange theory has something to say on this as well. It suggests that reward/cost balance alters due to changes in the person's characteristics, changes in any external circum-stances, ongoing aspects of the relationship, and associations with other behaviours which have different reward/cost outcomes. In this sense a relationship will endure over time as long as its outcomes are above the comparison levels which can be made for alternative relationships. This might be the case even when the two people are not that highly mutually attracted. It is just that the reward/cost balance they derive from their particular relationship is the best available to them at the time.

Overall then, it is clear that interpersonal attraction is a very important facet of person perception and the judgement of others. At present there are various theories to account for it, each of which has some support. Perhaps the best of these in that it seems to be the most far reaching, is exchange theory.

Summary Points

(1) Judgements and perceptions of other people are all based on inferences made from how they look and what they do. Techniques to study these processes in the laboratory need to be carefully checked as to their artificiality.

(2) First impressions are important unless a person is warned against them or unless they are followed by a gap in time and then further information.

(3) Some traits assume more importance in our judgements of others than do other traits. These are said to be central.

(4) The most important aspect of judgements about other people is concerned with the recognition of emotional expression. Of particular importance in this context is the question of whether emotional expressions depend on a few dimensions, the extent to which movement is involved, the relevance of the context in which the emotion is being expressed, the ways in which attempts are made to hide emotions and deceive others, and the extent to which emotional expression is innately determined and hence universal.

(5) Although important, the accuracy which people show in judging others is very difficult to assess. When it does appear that one person is more accurate than the next, this might be a spurious impression. One cannot yet say whether such accuracy is a general skill or what are the qualities of a good judge of personality or character.

(6) Of especial significance in the field of forming impressions of others is interpersonal attraction. There are various theories of this which lay stress on different aspects such as the person, personal needs, the interaction, and so on. The best of these seems to be social exchange theory which accounts for attraction in terms of reward/cost balances.

Study Questions – 13

(1) During the course of your day-to-day work it is inevitable that you make many judgements of the character and personality of your

patients. How do you do this? What do you take into account?

(2) How influential on your subsequent behaviour are the first impressions you make of a patient? Do you think that you should give much weight to first impressions?

(3) How much do you think you can judge about a patient from his: accent, clothes, hair, walk, shape of face, hands? Would such judgements alter the way in which you behaved towards him?

(4) How easy do you find it to judge what a patient feels emotionally about you or his treatment or his general circumstances from his facial expressions? To what extent do you need information other than facial expression to make such judgements?

(5) It is possible that some of your colleagues or those who have helped to train you are extremely good in their professional role partially because they are good judges of character and personality in their patients. If you agree with this, what qualities do you think these good judges of character possess? Could you develop them in yourself?

(6) Do you think that the impression of you that your patients have is similar to that which your colleagues have of you? What do you think are the major differences and why do you think they exist? Which of the two would have the more accurate impression?

(7) Think of instances in which you have radically changed your impression of a patient. What has caused you to revise your judgement?

(8) Do you think that people in general make particular types of judgement of character about those who are ill? What form do such stereotypes take? Do you think that there might be any truth in them?

(9) It is well known that people who have some form of obvious physical disability or handicap are judged very differently from those who are physically normal. How would you take this into account in your professional capacity?

(10) The relatively closed society of a hospital in which people are thrown together in their jobs is an obvious framework for the development of interpersonal attraction and dislike. From your observations, what are the main determinants of this? How can it best be dealt with so that it does not obtrude into your professional role?

14 LEARNING AND TRAINING SOCIAL SKILLS

It is possible to argue that one cannot interact with another person without being changed by the experience in some way, even though the change might be minimal and occur without awareness. Just as the forensic scientist works according to the maxim that a person *always* leaves a physical trace of himself on the environment, so the social psychologist might argue that the person always leaves a trace of himself on the social environment; also more important, the social environment leaves a trace on him. If people are changed by their social encounters, then it is reasonable to assume that they learn socially.

In the last chapter mention was made of Argyle's analysis of social behaviour by assuming that it is a skill which is somewhat akin to a motor skill. Up to a point it is clear that this viewpoint has some merit. If one goes along with it, then it becomes even more reasonable to think of people acquiring, learning, modifying and qualifying their social behaviour, largely of course as a result of their social encounters. In fact, social behaviour is one of the few (if not the only) human capacity which does not reach its maximum early in life and then slide gently downhill. Most people *seem* to show steady improvement in their social behaviour throughout their lives. (The word 'seem' is stressed here because this point is difficult to document precisely.)

Looking at the possible learning of social skills from another viewpoint for a moment, there are countless everyday examples of social incompetence. We have all suffered embarrassment at the hands of others, or in empathy with their embarrassment, or have even caused them embarrassment from time to time. People transgress interactional norms constantly. They do not look one another in the eye often enough, they only smile with their mouths and not their eyes as well, they interrupt conversations, they joke in the wrong context, they cannot end conversations, and so on. At such times the individual concerned *seems* to have learned not very much socially. However they must have learned an enormous amount to be able to interact at all. The various signs of incompetence which they show from time to time, or even habitually in some cases, do not reflect a lack of learning but rather the learning of socially inappropriate behaviour (for the particular culture).

In a much earlier chapter the question of socialisation in children was considered. It is obvious that children become socialised, to a greater or lesser extent. They must *learn* socially, and the attention of psychologists has been directed to *how* this learning occurs. However, what is often forgotten is that the socialisation process never really ends, although it might slow down considerably. It could be said to end with social *maturity*, but this is a concept which no one can define adequately in any case. Social interaction and hence socialisation changes constantly.

Thinking then, of adult socialisation, Argyle (1964) again, argues that there are three ways in which it comes about. Although these are fairly self-evident, they provide a reasonable frame of reference.

(1) Instrumental Learning. Social behaviour changes through the usual rewards and punishments, be they delivered in a conscious effort to change someone (parents bringing up children or behaviour therapists dealing with clients) or be they simply an un-thought-out part of social interaction.

(2) Perception and Interpretation. Concentrating on the cognitive side of things it is possible to see how adult socialisation might come about through changes in the way in which social events are perceived and interpreted. This might lead to changes in attitudes (see Chapter 15) and might also involve changes in self perception. Take for example the change in self-perception which occurs when wearing very formal clothes after usually wearing informal clothes.

(3) Arousal. Here Argyle is stressing social learning which has an obvious emotional component, the type of social learning which might occur when the individual is under extreme pressure. A good example might come from the changes in attitude and social behaviour which occur in the turmoil of adolescence.

In an everyday situation, it would be very unlikely that these three routes to social learning would be separable; they would be bound together. Think for instance of a person just taking up his or her first job. Apart from finishing off the learning of the skills and techniques of the job itself, he would also have to learn the appropriate social behaviours. He would have to learn how to speak to people in the same building, but in different roles from himself; he would have to learn what to wear; he might start to pick up new expressions, both verbal and non-verbal; he is being changed by, is learning through, the complex social situation in which he finds himself.

Arguably the best actual examples of the sort of processes just mentioned occur in large institutions such as hospitals which employ a variety of people in various occupations. They tend to be distinguished by the clothes they wear, their physical territory, the manner in which they speak to one another, and so on. All of which has to be learned by the novitiate.

Learning Roles

At some time or another almost everyone has to learn new roles. The behaviour expected of a child is different from that expected of an adult. The behaviour expected of a trainee in some occupation is different from that expected of the same person when qualified. Parents whose children have grown up and left home have to learn new roles; people have to learn new roles in their retirement, and so on.

Secord and Backman (1974) distinguish between the content and process sides of role learning and then make a thorough analysis of these.

What is Learned in Roles – Content

In order to become accepted within a new role a person has to learn the *norms and rules* which usually go with the role. Thus for example, to some extent a nurse has to share the attitudes of other nurses rather than those of doctors, or an occupational therapist has to share attitudes with others in the same role rather than with administrators. And so on. Even the retired person has to take on (albeit unwillingly in some cases) the attitudes of other retired persons. This is not to say that the learning of one new role rather than another leaves one unsympathetic to the other person's role (again thinking of the many hospital examples), but simply that the first priority is to learn the appropriate role. This has to be done in order to gain acceptance. A nurse, or indeed any person in the medical or paramedical professions who appears to panic in an emergency will not be easily accepted in the role of the job.

Second, acquiring a new role involves the learning of *new social skills.* The individual has to learn how to deal with other people who are in the same role as himself. Learning the social role of a student is a good example. Not only does a student need to acquire academic and practical knowledge he also has to learn how to cope with his fellow students. Since these come from many walks of life and are in a rather artificial situation the social learning required is somewhat difficult, and can lead to considerable strain.

Thirdly, the content side of role learning involves *identity*, according to Secord and Backman, although this aspect is perhaps rather more debatable. They argue that in a new role a person has to learn an *ideal* conception of himself in that role. So for example, a person who has just qualified as an occupational therapist, apart from anything else, has to acquire a picture of herself as she would ideally like to be in the profession within a few years. This is a picture that she can gradually work towards. Probably the way in which this is done is by emulating someone who is already successful in the profession and who is admired, much as a child tends to identify with and emulate an admired adult. Although this process no doubt does occur, whether or not it is *necessary* to the learning of a new role is debatable.

How Roles are Learned – Process

In most instances roles are not taught, rather they are actively acquired through practising, problem-solving, and observing the behaviour of others already in the role. Secord and Backman eludicate the process of role learning by considering the factors which might enhance or impede it.

The social system is probably the main influence on how roles are learned. And the main aspect of importance in the social system is the *rewards and costs* it has developed in association with the particular role. What will it cost a person to adopt a new role in comparison with what it will benefit him? Will the financial and security and status advantages of a particular job outweigh the penury and general inconvenience and hard work involved in studying for it for some years?

Also, roles differ with respect to how clearly they are *defined* by society. For example, the social role of a member of the professional staff in a hospital is much less clearly defined (and much more complex) than that of a member of the maintenance staff. In general it is more difficult to learn a role which is less clearly defined than to learn one which is more precisely defined. Related to this is the matter of *similarity* between the new role and any previous role which the person has learned. The more similar are the two roles, or at least the more compatible, the more easily will the new one be learned. And of course it is the social system which determines how similar any two roles might be. For example it would be easier for any member of any of the paramedical services to learn the roles involved in any of the other paramedical services than it would for him to learn the role of a civil servant.

Much of the way in which new roles are learned seems to depend on what has gone before, often in a person's *fantasy* life. The most common example of this is given by the person who works alongside his superior, whose job he would like to have. He probably spends considerable time in imagining to himself how he would do the job if he were given it, and would therefore find it easier to adopt the role if he were given it than would an outsider.

Finally the social system determines what is called the *pervasiveness* of a role, and this in turn influences its learning. If a role is very broad and covers many different aspects of life then it will be learned more slowly than if it were more circumscribed. For example it should take far longer to learn the complex roles of a social worker than it would to learn the roles of a worker on an assembly line.

The *situation* is the other main source of influence in the learning of social roles. That the situation can have an important effect here is best exemplified by those institutions which bear the point in mind and use it to their advantage. It is particularly important where fairly extreme changes have to be wrought.

Good examples come from institutions such as the armed forces. In dealing with new recruits such organisations tend first to *desocialise*; they cut off the person from his previous source of reward and punishment, from all previous roles. Then they attempt to build the person up in the new role. They do this constantly so that he has no time to think of anything else. All of his waking hours are spent within that role, and there are so many waking hours that he is too exhausted to do anything other than sleep when he goes to bed.

To some extent this process of resocialisation occurs in almost any institutional or organisational setting, even if it is not so overt as it might be in the forces. Any new member of a large group tends to be looked on (and made to look on himself) as the lowest of the low. He has no status and has unpleasant roles to fulfil, whilst the established member has enormous status and apparently much more pleasant roles. And he is allowed only to interact with the new group, or at least it is difficult not to. This all provides motivation for learning the new roles. The whole process is sometimes helped along by various rituals and ceremonies, almost like those involved in a wedding for example, after which the persons concerned are expected to have taken up their new roles.

In general it can be said, that not only children but adults learn new roles all the time, and that they do this in fantasy and reality. Of course the most important new roles they learn are those which involve a considerable change in status, such as getting a first job, getting married, having a family, and so on. However, in a more mundane sense, many new social situations will involve the learning of new roles. Role learning seems to be a continuous process which is basic to social learning in general.

Learning and Group Processes

There has not been a great deal of work which has looked at group processes from the viewpoint of social learning. This is a little surprising since it is obvious that membership of a new social group would lead to the learning of some new social skills. Some of the relevant ideas are considered in the next chapter in the section concerned with liking and disliking. For now, the idea of social reinforcement in a group setting will be explored.

Group social reinforcement promoting learning within the group is a complex matter. For example if person A is reinforced by the group through them giving him a higher status, not only will this affect his behaviour, but it might also affect B's and C's as well. By contrast it might be a punishment to them.

Homans (1961) makes an interesting analysis of these types of complexities. He dwells on *rewards*, i.e. whatever the individual receives from a social exchange, and *costs*, i.e. whatever the individual has to give up in the exchange. Costs might include any risks which he has to take socially. At face value this might seem a good way to view social interaction and to account for some of the social learning which occurs within a group. However, in the individual case, rewards and costs might be very difficult to identify, particularly if it is ongoing inter-action which is being analysed. Motivation for behaviour within a group is sometimes very surprising in not being what it appears.

Homans' central assumption is that any behaviour which A emits in response to B is *valued* by B, and that the more generally valuable A's behaviour is thought to be then the greater is the *esteem* in which he is held. If one now thinks of this applying to the whole group rather than just to one or two members, the final stage in the assumption may be seen. That is, the more valuable in general is the behaviour of all the members of the group to all the other members, then the more *cohesive* the group will be, the more it will hang together as a unified whole. A possible mechanism such as this will apply a constant pressure on the members of the group to increase their mutual attraction and the general cohesion within the group. Take for example the members of a team working together on some practical problem. The more they hold one another's contributions in high regard and come to rely on them, then the greater will be the general *esprit de corps* in the group and also probably the greater will be its efficiency.

Conformity

One of the most important ways in which group cohesiveness is affected by learning seems to be through conformity. Conformity has been defined as instrumental behaviour which is maintained through reinforcement. On the other hand it is possible to view conformity as a *reward* which promotes social exchanges between group members, or even as a sort of advance payment for rewards which might be received in the future. In general then, people are regarded as learning to conform to the norms and customs of their groups. They do this either through reinforcement which might be part and parcel of the behaviour itself (the pleasure in behaving like the others), through anticipated rewards (conform and be promoted), or through mutual attraction (birds of a feather flock together and their plumage becomes even more similar).

In recent years learning to conform to social customs has been shown to have two very unfortunate outcomes. It helps to determine what has been termed obedience to authority and the egocentric behaviour of the innocent bystander.

Milgram (1974) has worked on *obedience to authority*. He carried out a long series of investigations the basic format of which will be described. They involved asking a subject to come to a room in which there was a large machine apparently capable of delivering electric shocks to another person. The subject was given one or two mild shocks and then told that he would be able to use the machine to get another subject to learn something. When the second subject made a mistake he could shock him if he so wished. The second subject (a confederate of the experimenter) was supposedly sitting on the other side of the apparatus wired up to the shock machine.

Facing the real subject was a graded series of buttons purportedly representing a graded series of shocks that he could give, and he was encouraged to work up the grades if the person he was 'teaching' kept making mistakes. You might think that no one would agree to such conditions, but in fact most of Milgram's subjects did agree, many of them working right through all the levels of shock up to the (apparently) most severe. At times they would hear the gasp or cry from the next room as the other person was 'receiving' his shock. In one condition they were even told that the other person had a heart condition, but that he would probably be all right. Of course, even then the confederate subject always made a set number of mistakes, and the real subject would give him his electric shocks, in order to point out to him the error of his ways. In the extreme the confederate with the heart condition even became ominously quiet after a particularly severe shock. But with the experimenter's encouragement many of the real subjects still carried on giving even more intense shocks.

Milgram explains his rather horrifying results by suggesting that during the course of their upbringing his subjects (like all of us) had simply learned to be obedient to authority. They were ordinary people and the experimenter was a scientist in a white coat with a lot of complex apparatus, and he was 'telling' them what to do. Such, according to Milgram, it might have been in Nazi Germany. Be this as it may, people do seem to have learned to obey authority and there might well be times when this could have unpleasant effects.

No less pleasant are the results of the research into the behaviour of the *innocent bystander* (e.g. Darley and Latane, 1968). Here the basic type of experiment has been to stage an accident to a woman whilst she was surrounded by people completing questionnaires. When they were working alone, 70 per cent of the subjects offered to help the woman, but when working in pairs only 20 per cent did. This and many similar sorts of study show that people seem to learn to view non-intervention as an act of conformity. If you are seen to be in trouble by a group of people then you are *less* likely to receive help than if only one person sees your difficulties.

Nothing in social psychology is as simple as this of course, so there are exceptions to this general rule. Help tends to be given in a very crowded, enclosed environment, like a lift or a train, when the on-lookers are absolutely face to face with the victim. There is no escape from social involvement in a situation such as this. However, the general point is that not only do we learn to become obedient to authority but we also learn to become uninvolved, unless presumably we are told to become involved by someone in authority.

Teaching Social Skills

So far in this chapter only one point has been made in a number of different ways, and that is that everyone learns social skills, either in interaction with one other person or in broader group interaction. This being so, it is possible to turn the coin over and question whether or not it is possible to teach people social skills. This question can be answered at one level by a simple affirmative. Parents, wittingly or unwittingly, teach their children social skills constantly; therapists, whatever their persuasion, alter their patients' social skills markedly. But what of relatively normal adults? Is it possible to teach them to improve their social skills? and if so, how?

As usual it is Argyle (1969) who has made the systematically most useful contribution in answer to these questions. He argues that social competence has four main aspects, each of which can be trained. Before going onto particular training or teaching methods, it is worth mentioning these four aspects.

(1) Motivation. Here, Argyle is referring to a person's enduring personality traits, which he feels, although relatively long-lasting can be changed by training.

(2) Perception. This refers to perception of self and others in a social context, which Argyle thinks can be trained by making the person more aware of social subtleties and nuances.

(3) Responses. This is the obvious aspect. It should be possible to manipulate a person's social responses so that they are viewed as generally more adequate.

(4) Presentation. Finally, and perhaps more debatably, Argyle suggests that it might be possible to alter the way in which a person presents himself to the world, and therefore indirectly to alter his social behaviour.

There are four major ways in which the teaching of social skills occurs. Although their effectiveness has not been evaluated equally, each will be discussed in turn.

Everyday Learning

The everyday learning of social skills has been the main topic of discussion in this chapter so far. This is the most common way in which adults learn new social responses, even though they typically receive very little feedback for their responses, and they have even less formal training. As pointed out in the last chapter, Argyle lays great emphasis on the importance of feedback to this sort of 'natural' social learning, simply by analogy with other forms of learning. The problem is that it is difficult in most contexts for one adult to give another any direct social feedback. It is somehow like saying that he has bad breath or that he smells. To do this, one has to know the person extremely well or to have enormous power and influence over him.

There is little else one can say about the everyday learning of social skills, other than the preceding discussions in this chapter. Obviously, this is how much of the social learning of adults occurs, but it is a haphazard chancy business.

Formal Learning

Is it possible to teach social skills by the old formal system of lectures, discussions and films? Certainly, knowledge can be conveyed in this way, but there has been little research into the effectiveness of such methods in actually changing people's behaviour. Argyle feels that formal methods of instruction can affect social skills, but only when they are endorsed by other types of influence.

It is easy enough for an expert to lecture or to write about the subtleties of social behaviour and about what is involved in what can be termed a skilled social performance. It is very difficult to assess how effective this might be. Although an individual might say that he understands quite well what is being said, he may not change his behaviour because of it. The two major problems with formal instruction of social skills are that they will often be concerned with the teaching of non-verbal skills with verbal material, and they cannot really insist on practice at the skills themselves.

Role-playing

Knowledge concerning the ways in which new roles are learned in everyday life has been put to use in the training of people in various social capacities. The procedure which is usually followed is firstly to make up a list of problems which the person will have to face in the job or social situations for which he is being trained. Then incidents are constructed which have these problems at their core, and the person is put into these artificial situations and asked to play various roles within them. For example a prospective interviewer might be face-to-face with someone who never looks at him, or who talks too much, or who never seems to talk at all. Or for instance a person training to work in a hospital might be faced with a patient who is completely unco-operative or persistently negative.

Essentially then role-playing involves exercises in simulation. Inevitably they rest on one assumption, that is that the person running them knows what the problems of the particular job or situation are and knows what social skills are necessary to overcome them. Such an assumption may or may not be well founded in the individual case. Certainly there is no generally recognised list of social problems and skills as they pertain to various occupations.

Usually, whilst a person is playing out his various roles he is watched in this by the other people involved and a videotaped record is made of his performance. Afterwards, the videotape is played and analysed slowly, the person being given feedback as detailed as possible. Again, research into the effectiveness of this in the training of social skills is very scarce. However, Argyle is reasonably convinced that such methods have much to be said for them. Also, there are many other social psychologists who use role-playing techniques and videotapes who are convinced as to their effectiveness. The feedback aspect is perhaps the most important. This will be very clear to anyone who has seen him or herself on videotape; to begin with it is far far worse than first hearing one's own voice on a tape recorder.

One important aspect of role-playing is that it provides a situation in which it is perfectly acceptable to make social criticism; after all, the person is playing a role rather than being himself. Argyle argues that such exercises lead to increased social awareness and sensitivity, especially if the person has received strong negative feedback. However, this conclusion needs to be verified, and it is also important to take into account the difficulties involved in role-playing, particularly that the people concerned often feel it to be stupid and become very self-conscious. Also, there is the wide-open question of the extent to which it generalises from the laboratory or class-room to real life.

T (training) Groups

T groups (or sensitivity groups) are probably the most common way of trying to bring about social learning in adults at the moment. They are certainly in vogue. They fill a sort of hinterland between ordinary teaching and psychotherapy. The description which follows may be found in more detailed form in Argyle (1969) and Aronson (1976).

Those who run T groups have very grand aims. These are to:
(1) increase social sensitivity in general,
(2) develop a clearer perception of oneself,
(3) improve awareness of how others see oneself,
(4) learn to be accepting and yet independent,
(5) produce more effective work,
(6) learn how to learn socially.

The main principle which underlies the workings of T groups is that the members are to learn from one another by communication. This means that everything that is said is explored in great detail. In everyday life if someone says or does something, everyone around who is interested sees this and ascribes various motives to him and gives reasons for his behaviour, and then probably forgets it. The same procedure is followed in a T group but much more frankly and overtly. However, all that is discussed is what is going on at the time. The members of such groups do not have to reveal their long-term goals or fears or hopes, but to keep everything very much in the present.

As with all social learning, the emphasis on T groups is on feedback, The aim is to give everybody *immediate* feedback about whatever they say or do socially. What they do with this feedback is entirely up to them; it is perfectly open to them to reject it, but of course if they do this might be commented on as well. Clearly the giving of feedback in this type of situation is no easy matter, because too much honesty can be very hurtful. This particular problem is circumvented in a very cunning way. All the participants are encouraged to explore their *feelings.* For example, it is far easier to accept from someone the statement 'I feel that you are insincere' than it is to take the statement, 'You are insincere'. The point is that if it is honestly given, an expression of feelings is a factual statement which says something about he who says it as well as about he to whom it is directed. On the other hand the judgement involved in 'You are insincere' is mere conjecture but it is couched in such a way that it sounds very much like a fact.

As well as this the members of T groups are encouraged to try to work out one another's intentions. We all know people whose social style is such that they will say something *in such a way* that it will sound very hurtful, though they did not intend to be hurtful. If one is socially ill-at-ease to begin with, it is easy to assume that the hurt was meant.

T groups then are very intense and complex situations. How effective are they? For once in this area of the learning of social skills there have been a number of relevant research studies. However, these are rather difficult to evaluate, mainly because they lack some of the necessary control groups. Take an example. Typically, T groups are arranged such that the group comes together in a country house for a long week-end and whilst there the rules of sensitivity training apply. How can one separate the effects of the training from those of simply being in a country house for four days, or simply being away from home, or simply meeting a new group of people? In evaluating T groups it is very difficult if not altogether impossible to make comparisons with the appropriate control groups.

These limitations apart, some generalisations can be made. People who have experienced sensitivity training do seem to pay more attention to interpersonal matters, although their social perception is not necessarily improved. Human relationships do seem to be improved. However, against these general gains must be weighed the disadvan-

tages of T groups. Situations as intense as these must carry some
dangers with them. They put so much pressure on some people that
they break down; they cannot stand it. It is difficult to cope with
extreme and constant feedback, criticism and explorations of one's
feelings.

Argyle, in summary concludes that T groups benefit about 30-40 per
cent of their members but are of definite harm to others. Also he
suggests that as yet there is no firm evidence that they do teach social
competence. T groups members certainly learn socially, but this might
not be to their benefit and might not lead them to be more skilled
socially.

Theory

So far this chapter has contained little in the way of theory. This simply
reflects the state of affairs in this area of concern; there has not been
much theory. However, what does exist has been fairly influential and
so two representative theories will be discussed briefly.

Theoretical contributions began with Miller and Dollard (1941, 1950)
who applied Hullian learning theory to social behaviour. The corner-
stones of their theory were:

(1) *Drive* — which can be innate or acquired although in adult social
behaviour is normally acquired based on fear or money or approval, for
example. They argued that any stimulus can become a drive if it is
strong enough.

(2) *Cues* — again any strong stimulus can function as a cue and so determine when and where a person responds and what responses he makes.

(3) *Response* — which is self-evident, and is learned most easily if
followed by —

(4) *Rewards.*

In 1941 Miller and Dollard argued that much of social learning is
brought about by the secondary drive of anxiety and the secondary
reward of relief (from anxiety) which reduces the drive. So for example,
a person will learn a new social response (for example, to look at people
more often when he talks to them) in order to reduce or avoid the
anxiety which is caused to him by embarrassment. He is reinforced in
this by the relief from no longer feeling so anxious socially. Later on
Miller and Dollard became much less behavioural and spoke more in
terms of higher mental processes bringing about these changes in social
behaviour.

Homans' (1961) theory of social exchange has already been mentioned above. It is most easily summarised by mentioning its main vari-

ables and formal propositions. There are two main variables.

(1) *Value*. The value of a social act depends upon the degree of reinforcement and punishment associated with it. Values reflect individual preferences which themselves depend on the person's past history.

(2) *Quantity*. This is the number of units of activity performed within a given time. It is the Skinnerian idea of rate of response.

Homans' five propositions are as follows:

(1) Similarity — if a present stimulus situation is similar to one in the past in which there has been a reward for some social activity, then it is likely that the person will emit the same activity.

(2) Frequency —'the more often A's activity rewards B's activity then the more frequently B will behave in that way.

(3) Value — the more valuable is a unit of A's activity to B, then the more often B will produce the behaviour which leads to it.

(4) Reward — the more frequently B has recently received rewarding activity from B then the less value it is to him.

(5) Justice — the more a person sees a social situation as becoming unfair to himself, the angrier he will become.

It should be fairly evident by now that underlying all of these rather turgidly spelled out ideas, is the simple law of effect. Homans is arguing that we learn socially for profit, that is through our evaluations of profits against costs. It can be said that this highlights the difficulties of theory in social psychology. Even when taking a very rigorous behavioural approach as does Homans, it still seems necessary to end by speaking of an *evaluation* of profit and cost — a very non-behaviourist idea.

Conclusions

This chapter has attempted to give an idea of some of the work on social learning in adults and in the training of social skills. This is a difficult area about which to draw conclusions. It is obvious that we learn new social responses and modify old ones constantly. On the other hand most text-books of social psychology rarely mention such learning. They are more concerned with discrete topics such as group processes, attitudes and so on.

One can say that any aspect of social behaviour involves learning. The problem then becomes one of narrowing down any discussion to the most salient aspects. Such has been the aim of this chapter. Adults do learn social skills and can be trained to increase their social competence. However, a great deal more research needs to be done on how such learning occurs in an everyday context and on the most effective training methods.

Summary Points

(1) Everyone is changed by his or her social encounters and must therefore be learning from them. Individual differences in social competence
also point to this. Argyle argues that such learning comes about instrumentally, through perception and interpretations and through arousal.
(2) An important aspect of social learning involves the learning of new
roles. This can be broken down into its content, consisting of learning
rules, new social skills and an identity; and its process. The process of
role learning is influenced by the social system (through rewards and
costs, similarity between roles and pervasiveness of roles) and the situation in which it occurs.
(3) What people in groups learn socially seems to depend on an equation
between rewards and costs. Of particular importance here is mutual
attraction and liking which can ultimately lead a group to be very
cohesive; this is beneficial.
(4) Group cohesiveness is importantly affected by conformity. Two
rather disturbing aspects of conformity are the way in which people
have apparently learned to obey authority and also to remain uninvolved in a group situation when someone needs help.
(5) Social skills can be taught but the effectiveness of the various
teaching methods has not yet been assessed adequately. Much social
learning and teaching simply occurs as a part of everyday life. Also,
formal teaching methods can be used but seem unlikely to be very
effective. Role playing with feedback has its strong adherents, but of
especial importance these days is sensitivity training given in T groups.
Although these do bring about social learning, whether or not this
learning is always to the individual's advantage remains to be seen.
(6) Social learning theory has not gone very far even though it has been
around for many years. It occurs in both a Hullian and a Skinnerian
tradition but in either case cannot avoid mentalistic interpretations.

Study Questions – 14

(1) Describe as many examples as you can of social incompetence that
you have observed in your job (including your own). What has gone
wrong with social learning in these cases?
(2) What aspects of your own social behaviour do you think might irri-
tate different people? How could you alter such behaviour?

(3) Do patients in hospital have new social roles to learn? If so, what are they? What are their main characteristics?

(4) Do you play a different role or roles in your professional life than in your private life? What are the differences and how are they affected by the situations in which you find yourself?

(5) To what extent do you think that the processes of socialisation and resocialisation mentioned in this chapter have been employed in your own training and are applied to patients in hospitals?

(6) Hospitals tend to be arranged hierarchically and people within them expected to conform. Why do people conform and obey authority? Have you seen any examples of people in groups not helping those in difficulties? Why do you think that this sometimes happens?

(7) How would you teach a social skill to a patient? How would you assess the effectiveness of your method?

(8) Design some role-playing situations that would be relevant to your job and enact them with colleagues. What are the main social problems you would encounter professionally and how would you overcome them?

(9) Doubtless, some of your patients and colleagues are less socially competent than others. Do you think that it would be possible to change them to be more socially acceptable? Would it be possible to train anybody to be completely at ease in any social setting?

(10) What changes in social competence result from illness and disability? Do you think that people in general tolerate more social incompetence from the ill and the disabled? If so, should they?

15 ATTITUDES AND PREJUDICE

The Objects and Components of Attitudes

It is self-evident that the assessment of attitudes has become an important industry in western society. There are public opinion polls, political attitude questionnaires, government surveys and market research companies who assess people's reactions to new packaging, new consumer items, and so on. The reasons for this interest in the attitudes of other people is equally self-evident. The aim, like some of those of psychology in general is to predict and therefore control behaviour. If it is found that most people within a certain income bracket in a particular town prefer brand X packaged in green paper then the manufacturers can package it that way and hence sell more of it. They have predicted and controlled behaviour through an assessment of attitudes. Similarly, if the members of a minority group in society know the attitudes of the majority towards them they will be better able to do something about possible aggressive acts.

The Objects

Because objects exist does not of course mean that everyone will have attitudes towards them. It is difficult to hold an attitude about an item which one has never seen. So an attitude is held towards any object which exists for the individual; he will therefore have a vast range of attitudes on all manner of subjects. However the range of his attitudes is limited by what may be called his psychological world. For example, not everyone living in a cosmopolitan area will have an attitude towards integration or segregation of the races. Similarly, not everyone working in a hospital will have an attitude towards a certain type of treatment for a particular disorder. It depends on their interests and concerns.

The Components

Psychologists regard attitudes as being made up of three components:
(1) a cognitive, or belief component
(2) an emotional or feeling component, and
(3) an action component.
Take for example the attitude a person might hold against organised religion. He might *believe* that it is degrading and only enjoyed by unthinking people; he might *feel* negative emotions whenever he saw it

going on; and he might have strong tendencies to behave in ways which impeded it, by arguing against it when the opportunity presented itself, for example.

The *cognitive* components of an attitude then are concerned with the beliefs which the individual holds. The most important of these are the *evaluative* beliefs, which involve the attribution of 'good' or 'bad' qualities to the object of the attitude. Also included here may be beliefs about appropriate and inappropriate ways of behaving towards it. It is the belief component of an attitude that those who assess attitudes are most concerned with. It is the most readily measured by means of question and answer.

The *emotional* component of attitudes is the aspect which gives them their rather stirred up and subjectively important character. The object of the attitude is felt as either pleasing or displeasing, it is liked or it is disliked. The feeling components of attitudes can be measured physiologically by indirect psycho-physiological techniques for assessing heart rate, respiration, the electrical conductivity of the skin and so on. Clearly though this requires laboratory equipment and is therefore only of academic rather than practical interest.

The *action* component of an attitude refers to what might be called the behavioural readiness which is associated with it. If a person holds a positive attitude towards something then he will feel disposed to spend time with it, seek it out, aid it, or whatever behaviour might be appropriate. If his attitude is negative he will be moved to harm, punish or even destroy it. So, if you are pro-black you might seek out blacks, help them and treat them as friends. Whereas if you are anti-black you might avoid them, reject them as friends, and treat them as inferiors. Often however a mildly held attitude will not result in any action at all, unless the individual is pushed into an extreme. For example many people have definite attitudes of sympathy to the many people in the world who have insufficient to eat, but few of them actually do anything about it.

Characteristics of Attitude Components

The three components of attitudes can vary along two important dimensions. The first is *valence*. Usually it is a simple matter to describe whether an individual's attitude is positive or negative, but it is often felt to be important to specify the degree of its direction. This is the valence of an attitude and applies equally to each of the three components. Thus one can believe something to be anything from extremely good to extremely bad, one can give it anything from unconditional love to unconditional hate, and one can have extreme tendencies to help and support to extreme tendencies to harm and destroy. It is the valence of attitudes with which those who attempt measurement are most concerned.

The second important component of attitude is their *multiplexity*. This simply refers to the range, variety and number of parts which make up the attitude and again is relevant to each of the three components. The cognitive component can be made up of a single belief about the object or can be based on a very complete knowledge of it. For example a Christian attitude may be based on a single belief in God and the existence of Christ, or may be the very complex set of beliefs based on Christian philosophy which might be held by a minister of the church.

Similarly, the feeling component of an attitude can vary from mildy positive or mildly negative to a very highly complex set of emotions. Compare for instance the relatively simple act of liking someone whom you have met for ten minutes to the love which you might feel for a member of your family. Also the action tendency can vary from a single positive or negative desire to a very highly elaborated set of be-haviours. Compare for example the single vote which someone might cast in a general election with the very complex behaviour of the poli-tician for whom he might be voting. They both have a positive political attitude in a particular direction, but the behaviour of one is far more complex than that of the other.

Attitude Groups

So far discussion has centred on any one of an individual's attitudes; this will normally be the concern of the attitude measurer, he will not often try to assess more than one attitude at a time. It would be too difficult. But people hold complete sets of attitudes about which the question is often asked: how far are an individual's attitudes inter-connected?

As might be expected, attitudes differ with respect to how much they are related to other attitudes. For example, a person may be very keen to own his own house, but this attitude may be quite distinct from the remainder of what might be called his political attitudes which are very left wing and averse to general private enterprise and owner-ship. On the other hand his positive attitude towards the catholic religion might be closely related to his attitudes towards a whole range of objects — art, science, family relationships, birth control, and so on.

Except in the most bizarre individual, few attitudes will stand com-pletely alone, they will be related to some others. Sometimes the degree to which a person's attitudes form an orderly, coherent pattern is taken as an index of the extent to which his personality is unified, or perhaps even lacking in complexity. Although it (perhaps fortunately) is not possible to find a completely consistent individual, it does seem that most attitudes fall into three main clusters, at least according to one type of break-down. These three areas are: (1) religious – patterns of attitudes towards topics such as evolution, God, birth control, etc. (2) humanitarian – patterns of attitudes towards capital punishment, corporal punishment, the treatment of criminals, war, and so on; and (3) nationalism – attitudes towards politics, law, censorship, patriotism, and so on. It should be remembered that these are only rough categories under general headings which are a little arbitrary.

Attitude Measurement

Attitude measurement is an extremely complex and highly technical subject which will only be dealt with briefly. The normal way of assessing attitudes is to devise a scale consisting of a number of items which are specifically designed to tap attitudes towards the object in question. Just as with a personality scale the individual's scores on the attitude scale can then be compared with those of other people and his general position relative to theirs arrived at.

The difficulty in attitude measurement comes in the methods which are used to devise the scales. One fairly simple example can be seen with the *Likert scale*. In this a set of statements are made up which are pertinent to the attitude in question. To each item a series of judges have to indicate whether they: strongly agree, agree, are undecided, disagree, strongly disagree. The item might be for example, all Jews are shrewd rather than wise. Weights of 1, 2, 3, 4 and 5 are given to these responses in inverse order to agreement; so a strongly disagreeing response scores highly. The total score is then the sum of the weights for each response made to the series of statements.

This is just a beginning. At first many items are used. These are then reduced to a reasonable number by an *internal consistency analysis*. The extent is calculated to which the responses of the group to a particular item are consistent with the total scores on the scale. Any which are inconsistent are dropped. In practice those items are retained which best differentiate between persons with high or low total scores. Enough of these complexities; the Likert scale is one of the simplest.

Of particular importance in attitude measurement is what is termed the *neutral region*. This is the central area of an attitude scale which represents what appears to be the absence of an attitude one way or the other. It is an important area since those who measure attitudes would like to determine to which side of an exact central point a person falls. The argument is that if this can be ascertained then it would be possible to predict which way a person would jump if he were pushed into an extreme position in which he would have to make up his mind. However, most attitude scales are not very efficient at accurate definition of the neutral region. Perhaps this is not surprising since it is asking a lot to be able to make precise behavioural predictions from relatively insensitive questions and answers.

Attitude Changes

The topic of how attitudes change and can be changed is very large and has had a great deal of research effort poured into it. It can be divided broadly into two main aspects. First there is a tradition of building theoretical models of how the attitude change process might come about, and second there is an analysis of the sort of influences which are important in the changing of attitudes. These will be dealt with in turn.

Cognitive Dissonance

There are a number of theoretical models of attitude change of which the most interesting was proposed by Festinger (1957) and is known as dissonance theory. As a general caveat it should be said that although this theory is very beguiling it has a weakness that it explains so much that it is very difficult to use in order to make precise predictions.

The basic argument is that all of us seek *consistency* in our own behaviour and in those around us. *Dissonance* refers to a relationship between two things which is inharmonious, discrepant or inconsistent. *Cognitive dissonance* occurs when two cognitions or beliefs which a person holds are obviously inconsistent with each other according to the person's previous expectations based on his past experience. For example it would be dissonant if you lost your temper with someone and hit him, and he neither flinched nor hit back nor ran away.

The central hypothesis of cognitive dissonance theory is that the presence of dissonance produces a pressure to reduce the dissonance, the strength of this pressure being a direct function of the magnitude of the dissonance — the greater the dissonance, the stronger the pressure to do something about it.

Cognitive dissonance can be reduced in one of three ways, each of which would represent a change in the person's attitudes. This is best illustrated with an example.

Cognitive dissonance: 'I smoke and yet believe that smoking causes lung cancer and various bronchial complaints.'
I can reduce this dissonance by:
(1) Changing one or more of my cognitions to bring them into line. Thus I could stop smoking, or perhaps stop reading about and listening to reports of the relationship between smoking and disease.
(2) Adding new cognitions which strengthen one or other side of the two dissonant cognitions. Thus I might say, 'All my friends smoke and none of them have lung cancer; it must be all right.'
(3) Decreasing the subjective importance of the whole matter. Thus, I might say, 'You've got to go sometime; it might as well be by smoking as anything else.'

The weakness of dissonance theory is that although it provides a neat way of outlining the forces for attitude change and suggests ways in which this might come about, it does not allow any assessment to be made of which way will be chosen in the individual case.

Persuasion

Persausion is an attempt to change people's attitudes and as such may be seen as an integral part of everyday life. It is but a short step from this to politics, religion, education, and even indoctrination. It is therefore important to determine how persuasion works. According to Aronson (1972) for example, there are three important factors which help to determine persuasibility: the nature of the message designed to persuade, where it comes from and to whom it is directed.
(1) *The nature of the message* has four important aspects. (a) It can be expressed in logical or emotional language. In general it is more effective in bringing about change if it is emotional, particularly if it makes a person relatively anxious to begin with and then shows him how a change in his attitude will reduce the anxiety.
(b) It is possible to present both sides of an argument or just one. Here, effectiveness depends on audience. A more intelligent audience is more likely to be persuaded by a two-sided communication and a less intelligent by a one-sided.
(c) Information can be presented in a number of different orders. In general it is best to present the most important item *first* if the other information is to follow on immediately and if the audience does not have to make a decision for some days. However, if there is a time gap between the bits of information and a decision has to be made immediately, then it is best to have the most important item last.

(d) Should the message be extreme or mild? Some psychologists argue that this depends on the source of the information. If this is highly credible then the message can be extreme and still effective. If the source is less then it is best that his message is not too discrepant from the existing views of those he is setting out to persuade.

(2) Of major importance in the *source* of a message is its *credibility*. Information from a high status source such as *The Times* rather than the *Mirror* or a leading sportsman rather than an unknown athlete is more likely to persuade. Linked to this is the *trustworthiness* of the source. Oddly enough for example a person in an attractive occupation will appear more trustworthy and hence more effective in changing attitudes than someone in a less attractive occupation. So, for instance, an athlete will make more people buy a breakfast cereal than will a nutritionist.

(3) Finally, there are features of the audience which are important in attitude change and persuasibility. In general, women are more easily persuadable than men, and a person who feels inadequate changes his attitudes more easily than one who enjoys high self-esteem. Also, a person will be more receptive to change if he comes to the situation in a relaxed, well-fed, content state.

Overall then if you want to change someone's attitude or persuade them of something you need to be of high status, to be credible and trustworthy; you need to take into account your audience, balance your words appropriately between the emotional and the logical, present information in the right order and with the right amount of discrepancy between yourself and the audience. Even then a person whose basic beliefs are being questioned tends to switch off and stop taking in information. In general, attitudes which have a firm emotional base are more difficult to change than those which have not. As will be seen below such is the case particularly with prejudice.

Prejudice and Discrimination

It is best to begin a discussion of prejudice with three important definitions.

(1) *Prejudice*, as the term implies is an attitude based on a pre-judgement; it predisposes a person to think, feel and behave in favourable (prejudice can be positive) or unfavourable ways to a group of its members. As with all attitudes, behaviour may follow although not necessarily. Prejudice is extremely resistant to change.

(2) *Stereotyping* is viewing the members of some group as having traits which distinguish them from the general population. It has three main

characteristics. (a) people are categorised according to some characteristics which identify them. For example someone might categorise a
group as university students. (b) People holding the stereotype agree on
certain attributes possessed by *all* people in the group. For example, all
students are long-haired and irresponsible. (c) There is a discrepancy
between the attributed traits and the actual traits. Of course, not all
students are long-haired and irresponsible any more than all Germans
have no sense of humour or all Italians pinch bottoms.
(3) *Discrimination* is the differential treatment of individuals who
belong to a particular social or cultural group; it is the overt behavioural
expression of prejudice and usually involves denying or granting the
individuals some right or privileges. Thus the membership of a club or
a profession might be restricted, for example.

A prejudiced attitude then involves prejudgement, tends to be based
on stereotyping and if it is expressed takes the form of discrimination.
The analysis of prejudice which follows can be found in more extended
form in Secord and Backman (1974).

Beginnings of Prejudice

The origins of prejudice (which for the purposes of this discussion will
be restricted to racial prejudice) are far more difficult to determine
than are the factors which help to maintain prejudice once it is established. However, usually two groups of people are involved with definite
differences between them in status and power. This social structure
seems to promote judgements which are consistent with it. Thus for
example, because of their much weaker social position blacks in some
parts of the world might come to be thought of as irresponsible and
lazy. Not only does this 'explain' the differences in status, it is also true
to say that *because* of the status differences the black might be unable
to demonstrate responsibility and industriousness.

Secondly, it has been shown that if a person is seen as having a very
different status than one's own, then he is also seen as having different
beliefs. Perceived differences in beliefs always tend to make people
edgy and therefore to promote prejudice.

Prejudice appears to develop in children just before they go to
school or at least in the early school years. In a mixed racial community
all children of whatever race show preferences for mixing with those
children from the majority group. Thus in a society which is racially
prejudiced against blacks, even the black children, when young, will
prefer to associate with white children. The objects of children's prejudices not surprisingly are those which prevail in the adult society, and

they tend to become aware of them at about 12 or 13. The prejudice develops directly from socialisation. The children simply learn the beliefs of their parents and so prejudice is perpetuated from one generation to the next.

The Maintenance of Prejudice

The factors which maintain racial prejudice can be broken down into three main groups, those which come from individual personality, those which come from the social structure, and those which come from the general cultural background.

(1) Individual Factors. There are at least four individual factors in the maintenance of prejudice which are worth mentioning. Perhaps the most important of these involves *frustration* and *aggression* and has given rise to the *scapegoating* theory of prejudice. There is a great deal of evidence in psychology that one of the most consistent outcomes of frustration is aggression. Sometimes, when the true source of the frustration cannot be retaliated against, the frustrated individual may turn on an innocent weaker party. The extreme of this is perhaps seen when a person who is frustrated in a family argument stalks out and slams a door or starts banging the pots and pans around, or kicks a chair. At a broader level in society it will very often be the innocent members of some minority group who are turned on.

If for example, an individual feels that he would like to work but cannot find a job, he is really being frustrated by the general society in which he lives. Or if he works but feels that he has to give too much of his money back to the government in taxes, he is being frustrated by the government. In either case there is not much that he can do, so he may turn on the members of the minority group who live in his area and misplace the blame for his frustration onto them. 'If they were not here I could get a job or I would pay less taxes because they wouldn't need supporting,' and so on. Of course the true basis of the frustration is not removed in this way, and so the hostility is likely to continue. Prejudice has resulted from a sort of scapegoating.

One of the best studies on this concerned anti-Semitic attitudes. Four groups of subjects were chosen, two scoring highly on an anti-Semitism scale and two with low scores. One of each of these groups was put into a situation which would arouse aggression (the experimenter insulted them); the other groups had the same experiences but without the aggression. All of the groups then were shown two sketches each containing four different males, two of whom had Jewish sounding names.

They made up stories about these pictures and the stories were scored afterwards for their aggressive content. The highly anti-Semitic subjects were more aggressive to the Jewish characters than to the others and there were no differences between the high and low anti-Semitic groups in their aggression towards the non-Jewish characters. It seems from this study that if a person is anti-Semitic and is frustrated then he may well have a tendency to displace his aggression towards Jews, although not towards other people.

A second individual point which is thought to maintain prejudice is the questions of *economics* and *status*. Although less well documented, it does seem to be the case that in those areas of society in which economic competition is most severe and in which status is shakier and more easily threatened, then prejudice seems to be the greatest. Thus typically there is more prejudice at the low end of society and in those areas in which some equivalent of 'keeping up with the Joneses' is an important aspect of life.

Thirdly, prejudice often seems to be the reflection of particular aspects of personality. There are many of these which can influence prejudice and there would be little point in listing them here. But for example, a personal need for status might be supported by prejudice if it allowed the person to see the members of the other group as of inferior status to himself. Or a need for security might be met by joining together with others in order to reject the members of some other group.

In a little more detail, one interesting factor of personality which can influence prejudice is *intolerance for ambiguity*. People range from those who see the world in completely black or white terms to those who see shades of grey everywhere and are rarely disturbed by uncertain situations. Generally, those who are more intolerant of ambiguity are more likely to be prejudiced. It may be that the prejudice helps to explain an ambiguous situation. I want to work but cannot get a job; it is because all these foreigners have come to my country and taken jobs which are rightfully mine. They should be kicked out.

Finally, there is the question of dissimilarities in beliefs, a matter that was mentioned earlier. One study which bore on this presented subjects with a series of pairs of descriptive statements about people; in some of these race was varied, in some belief was varied, and in some both was varied. The subjects had to indicate the extent to which they thought they could be friendly with the people. For example:
A white person who believes in God.
A black person who believes in God.

A white person who believes in God.
A white person who is an atheist.
In general, similarity of belief was found to be far more important than
similarity in race. It will probably be the case that if a person sees
another as having some characteristic very different from his own, such
as skin colour for example, then he may well perceive him as having
different beliefs which will foster prejudice. This is perhaps even likely
to be the case if he sees him as having different customs, such as eating
different foods at different times of the day, or even going to church on
the 'wrong' day of the week.

(2) The social structure. Again, when considering the social structure
there are four main sources of influence on the maintenance of prejudice. The first concerns *conformity*. Once prejudice and discrimination
have become part of the society the attitudes involved tend to
become normative; that is the members of the prejudiced group expect
one another to hold the attitudes. Also, if one of the group members
does not conform this would have its costs to him; he would probably
be ostracised if he persisted in his non-conformity.

A study carried out in South Africa bore on this source of influence.
The investigator divided white South Africans into high and low scorers
on a questionnaire designed to measure their degree of prejudice against
black South Africans. He also measured their general conformity to
social norms quite independently of prejudice. Those in the highly
prejudiced group were also much more socially conforming. It would
seem reasonable to conclude from this and from similar findings in the
southern states of America, that those people who are most likely to
conform to their society's norms are the most likely to be prejudiced.
Conformity and prejudice are related although it is not possible to be
certain of the direction of the causal linkages.

The second factor from the social structure concerns *patterns of
interaction*. Prejudice and discrimination create patterns of interaction
which increase the degree to which the prejudiced group coheres; this
in turn gives the group added strength. At the simplest level, the members of the group interact more with one another than they do with
members of the outgroup, which in itself will produce more positive
intragroup feelings and lead to greater cohesion.

Linked to this is the fact that the members of social groups tend to
look to one another for economic and social support. They reinforce
one another's basic beliefs and attitudes, including prejudiced attitudes,
which of course leads them into situations in which there is even more

pressure to conform to the group norms.

Thirdly, there is *leadership*. All groups have their leaders, either ascribed or achieved and these leaders tend to support the norms of prejudice and discrimination. People who emerge as leaders or who are elected as leaders, apart from many other characteristics, tend to be those who most centrally reflect the prevailing climate of opinion in the group. This is particularly the case with broadly based political leaders in society. If one of the prevailing opinions in the society is towards prejudice then prejudiced leaders will tend to emerge. Because they are leaders then they will help to promulgate the prejudiced attitudes.

Finally, the social structure provides supports for prejudice which come from the general *environment*. When prejudice has existed in a society for some time, the attitudes which it embodies tend to become normative in that society. Probably the best example of this can be seen in the attitude towards segregation in the southern states of the USA until recently, or in the attitudes towards segregation in South Africa currently. The attitudes become so much a part of the society that they become part of its social institutions.

Images of minority groups tend to become presented in the literature and other mass media of the society and endorse prejudice. Consider for example the manner in which the American Negro was portrayed in early films from Hollywood. More often than not he was seen as a fun-loving, not very bright, eye-ball-rolling, singing coon. When prejudice goes this far in a society, it may lead to certain of the *objective* aspects of the minority groups becoming consistent with the prejudiced attributes. So, for example, in many parts of the world, blacks do have less pay, live in worse homes and have less opportunity to behave as responsible members of the society; they have no choice in this.

(3) The culture. The final aspect of the maintenance of prejudice comes from the most broadly based influence of all — the culture. It was pointed out earlier how the socialisation process is important in the development of prejudice. This of course is a cultural factor since child upbringing is a matter which is largely determined by social influences. However, also of importance in this context is the relationship between culturally shaped *values* and prejudice.

In the most extreme examples of prejudiced societies, attitudes towards minority (so-called, even if they might be in the numerical majority) eventually become part of the cultural ideology. For example, *some* white South Africans *genuinely* believe blacks to be apelike, primitive and biologically inferior to themselves. Associated with this they will believe them to be violent and oversexed, and of course believe that mixtures between the races are thoroughly undesirable. Beliefs such as these provide a way of making an inconsistent set of attitudes, consistent, or in other words of reducing cognitive dissonance. So, in the extreme, one could believe in equal rights for all human beings and still be prejudiced against and hence discriminate against Negroes. If in some sense they are believed to be sub-human, then to discriminate against them is not to be inconsistent with a belief in basic equality of rights and opportunities for all *humans*.

Changing Prejudice

Attitude change was discussed earlier, and it is clear that attitudes do change and a reasonable amount is known about how this occurs and how to bring it about. However, it is quite clear that the general rules of attitude change and persuasion do not hold when it comes to prejudice. Prejudiced attitudes are extremely resistant to change and they certainly cannot be changed to any great extent by trying to persuade people. The only technique, if it can be called that, which works is that of *enforced* contact. This has been studied in three ways.

Some studies have been made of the *fighting services*, particularly the army in which there has been enforced contact between Negro and white soldiers. In one study, Negro volunteers were drafted into previously all white platoons. Attitude surveys were made before and after this. Beforehand, the surveyers showed that most of the white enlisted men and about two-thirds of the officers were against the integration. Two months after the drafting, it was shown that nearly 80 per cent of the white officers were more favourable to mixed companies and that more than 80 per cent of the men thought that the blacks made good combat soldiers and that the blacks and whites were interacting well. However, when the fighting was finished and the platoons broke up, for the most part the blacks and whites went their own ways.

Even less effective in bringing about long-term changes in prejudiced attitudes are enforced contacts through a person's *occupation*. For example in a number of large cities such as London or New York in which there is anti-Semitic feeling, it is often the case that Jews and Gentiles have to work side by side. The two groups get along perfectly well during the working day but there is no longer term change in attitudes. This is even known in New York as the five o'clock shadow. Jews and Gentiles go their own ways after work; they would not think of inviting one another to their respective homes. Of course, this is a very general statement to which there will be large numbers of exceptions. However, the broad point holds true; namely, that contact between prejudiced groups because of the work situation does not seem to bring about any lasting changes in attitude.

The most effective way in which prejudice seems to be changed is through enforced contact in *housing*. One study which was carried out on this interviewed samples of white and black housewives who had formed part of new housing projects, some aimed at integrated living and others aimed at segregated living (in the USA). Beforehand there were roughly equal amounts of prejudice in the various groups. After living in the new conditions for some time, the integrated projects had led to far more in the development of intimate personal relationships between Negroes and whites than had the segregated; at least the housewives concerned had become far less prejudiced than they had been.

The authors of this study sum up their work by saying that prejudice is likely to be lessened when people are put into situations where contact is compelled between them and the objects of their prejudice, given that three conditions obtain. 1) The behaviour of the objects of the prejudice does not conform to the prejudiced beliefs of the prejudiced group. If it did, then of course the attitudes would no longer be prejudiced; they would be quite reasonable. 2) The intimacy and amount of contact are sufficiently compelling. 3) The prejudiced individuals have other values or sources of influence which would not allow them to maintain prejudiced attitudes in the face of absolutely clear evidence that they are wrong. In practice what happens in living areas is that the people concerned most often make friends with their next door neighbours or with whoever happens to live opposite them. As distance increases so the likelihood of friendships forming decreases. So if Negroes and whites are thoroughly mixed up in this way the normal geographical influences on friendship patterns help to outweigh any reticence brought about by prejudice, and the prejudice begins to decrease as more accurate information about the people in the other group inevitably becomes available.

Summary Points

(1) The object of an attitude can be anything which is in the psychological world of the individual.

(2) Attitudes have three components: cognitive, emotional and behavioural. These can vary with respect to their valence (extent of their direction) and multiplexity (the number of elements which comprise them).

(3) A person's attitudes vary with respect to how well they form a connected whole. Those of most people tend to fall into major groupings.

(4) Attitude measurement is a difficult matter and is mostly accomplished by means of questionnaires or attitude scales, the construction of which is highly technical. Of particular importance is the neutral or central region of apparent indecision.

(5) There are various models of attitude change of which the best known is cognitive dissonance, which suggests that if a person has two beliefs which are inconsistent with each other this produces a force for him to do something about it. Although compelling, dissonance theory does not allow precise prediction.

(6) The use of persuasion as a technique of attitude change is best done bearing in mind relevant aspects of the message designed to bring about the change, the nature of the source of the message, and the nature of the audience, all of which interact in complex ways.

(7) A prejudiced attitude is based on a pre-judgement, stems from stereotyping and has its expression in discrimination.

(8) The origins of racial prejudice are difficult to determine but are related to status and socialisation. Various factors maintain racial prejudice and come from the influences of personality, the social structure and the general culture.

(9) Prejudiced attitudes are very resistant to change, although this can be best achieved by enforced contact between members of the two groups, particularly if the contact is long-lasting and compelling.

Study Questions – 15

(1) Make a description of your own attitudes towards your occupation and training and compare them with those of someone you know well. How consistent are they? Do they fall into patterns? How strongly are they held? Do you hold any attitudes which you would not think of expressing in behaviour? What would make you express such attitudes?

(2) Do people's attitudes change, (a) when they go into hospital, (b) when they are serious ill, (c) after they have been seriously ill, (d) when they have had an accident, and (e) if they are disabled?

(3) Describe some examples of cognitive dissonance you have seen in your patients. Do they produce a force for change? How do the changes occur?

(4) Are there any differences in the attitudes held by young and old patients? Do you think that attitudes change with increasing experience?

(5) Do you find that some of your patients and colleagues are more resistant to changing their attitudes than others? What makes them more resistant?

(6) Do you hold different attitudes towards patients who are of a different race from your own? Do these attitudes reflect national stereotypes? Do they affect your work? How would you combat them?

(7) Have you seen any examples of racial prejudice in your training and work? What purpose has been served by such prejudice? Have patients suffered as a result of it? How can such prejudice be guarded against?

(8) Are there any prejudices and stereotypes that people hold about hospitals and members of the paramedical services? What could be done about dispelling them?

(9) How would you set about changing a patient's attitude towards, (a) his illness or treatment, (b) irksome hospital rules and regulations, (c) the degree to which he has to be dependent on others?

(10) Do you find that your private and personal attitudes differ at all from those that you hold in your professional role? What are the differences and why do you think that they have developed?

16 LEADERSHIP AND GROUPS

This chapter is primarily about leadership and its types, styles, functions and determinants. However leaders are only ascribed to, or emerge in, groups. Without followers there can be no leaders. When studying leadership, it is therefore important to know something of the structure and functions of groups. A consideration of leadership can itself provide reasonable insights into group functions, but it will be helpful in the discussion which follows if some groundwork is laid concerning the structure of groups.

The Structure of Human Groups

A group can be defined as two or more persons in a state of social interaction, be this broad physical action or subtle communication. Usually, the members of a group share similar goals, and usually derive some pleasure from the joint activity. If a group continues for some time and remains centred round the solution of a particular set of problems (of work, leisure or whatever) then a structure will begin to emerge for the group. This structure will take the form of different roles and statuses for the group members; a division of labour in which the members do their particular jobs and receive various rewards for this. Many groups in society have such differentiated roles and statuses laid down by a long tradition, the groups have existed for so long (e.g. schools, the forces, large industrial concerns, professional sports clubs). Those who join such groups therefore become assigned automatically to roles and their attendant statuses.

Primary Groups

Primary groups are characterised by face-to-face interaction. They tend to fulfil a wide range of needs and desires for their members and to meet in a particular place. Probably the best and most universal example of a primary social group is the *family*, whether this be as it is known in western society or of some other form as may be found in more primitive societies. The family is the first primary group with which most people have contact, and it is also the longest lived.

Other examples of primary groups are those based on friendship or the selection of a mate. Again these are obviously based on intimate face-to-face relationships. Also, there are primary groups in which the contacts are less intimate although still face-to-face, based on shared interests such as the pursuit of some sport of leisure-time activity for example. Quite commonly such groups are also based on similarities in age, as might be the case with childhood or adolescent gangs, or social clubs for the over-sixties.

Secondary Groups

Secondary groups are formed far more deliberately than primary groups and tend to be based on conscious choices made on the basis of particular interests and needs. Although they might involve face-to-face contact, they do not depend on it. For example, political organisations, trade unions, or religious organisations are secondary groups. Many of the members of such groups may never meet. Probably their most important single feature is that there is usually training and education for specific skills for some of the group members.

Both primary and secondary groups may be stable or may be impermanent. For example, the major political parties in Britain represent relatively permanent secondary groups, whereas some of the minor parties which spring up from time to time are impermanent. Similarly, most families are relatively stable primary groups, although some break up quite rapidly and hence exemplify impermanence.

Group Characteristics

The major characteristics of groups will be discussed only briefly at this point since this is a topic which forms an important part of the analysis of leadership which follows. It should be remembered that the main principles which will be described have been gleaned from many hundreds of studies of groups each of which has certain drawbacks. Some studies are based on observation of real-life groups and are therefore open to various biasses and imprecision. Other studies have been undertaken in the laboratory with artificially constructed and rather short-lived groups, which therefore may be unrepresentative of groups in everyday life. However, certain factors seem to be significant enough that they tend to emerge consistently in spite of these methodological limitations of the research.

(1) Formality. Groups can be structured formally or informally. A formal structure is one in which roles are firmly predetermined and remain independent of individual desires. Informal groups have self-made, flexible and unstable roles. However, groups may begin with an informal structure and as they remain over an extended period of time gradually

move in the direction of formal structure. So, a group of friends meet to share a common interest and as their meetings continue over time so they begin to see a need for group officers and co-ordinators and the formal structure begins to build up. An organisation such as the army is a good example of a very formally structured group in which there are a number of other groups based on common interests and which have informal structures.

(2) Causes. There are three major factors of importance in the emergence of group structure. (a) Individual motivation, which will help to determine the sort of roles which are set up and who assumes them. (b) Differences in abilities and temperament influence the assumption of roles and statuses. (c) The physical environment is also important. For example the structure of a child's playgroup might well be dependent on the sheer amount of space available for play.

(3) Power. Power is the relative effect that one person has on another with respect to altering his role or status. Clearly, in this light a leader is a person with more power than any other within the group, although as will be seen below there is far more to leadership than this. In formal groups, the power structure tends to follow a hierarchical pattern with roles and statuses definitely and clearly fixed. A has power over B who has power over C and so on. In informal groups, power is more unstable and flexible, with some people exercising it in some areas and not in others.

(4) Communication. The communication system varies with the size and organisation of the group. For example in large formal groups the communication system will tend to function through a specific chain of command, and in turn the chain of command will function through carefully laid down channels of communication. On the other hand, the communication patterns in small primary groups will alter according to the changing roles and statuses of the group members. As will be seen later the communication structure of a group has an important influence not only on patterns of leadership but also on the effectiveness of the group and the happiness of its members.

Definition of Leadership

Leadership is one of the terms with which psychology abounds, on which most people have views and yet which are notoriously difficult to pin down. Psychologists have produced many different views of leadership and what follows will be a representative selection of these. The material in the remainder of this chapter can be found in a much expanded form in Stogdill (1974).

The following have each been proposed as ways of defining leadership.

(1) Leaders *focus group processes.* This might simply be a person who has a high potential at whatever the group is doing and who therefore acts as an integrator. For example, in a group of people gathered at the roadside around a broken down car, the best mechanic will probably assume leadership.

(2) Leaders are those people with great *strength of personality.* They have large numbers of desirable (at least to the group) traits and exercise influence and social control through the prestige this brings them. This is is a definition of leadership as a question of one-way influence, ignoring group interactions.

(3) Leaders are those who can *induce compliance* most easily. Again this is one-way influence with leadership viewed as guiding and directing others to do whatever is wanted. The rights and privileges of group members are forgotten in such definitions. Related to this are those definitions which see leadership simply as an exercise of *influence.*

(4) Leadership is sometimes seen merely as an act of behaviour, behaviour which results in others acting in desired ways. Although this might seem objective it is really ducking out of the problem of definition altogether.

(5) Leaders are sometimes defined as *persuaders*, or inspirers. This stresses the making of sympathetic emotional appeals to lead, rather than exercising authority.

(6) Leadership has been defined in terms of the *power relationships* within a group. This makes a leader the person who exercises most force within a group whilst being able to offer maximum resistance to any force exerted on him. Thus viewing leadership as the *relative* exercise of influence, a leader being more successful at it than his group members.

(7) Leadership can be defined as the means to *achieving group goals* or aims. This is a view which suggests that leaders integrate the objective of groups and the roles of group members.

(8) Sometimes leadership has been viewed as an *effect* rather than a cause. It is simply a status which grows out of interaction between the individual who becomes the leader and the remainder of the group. This is a very passive definition and probably only has meaning in situations in which the leadership is recognised and conferred on the individual by the group.

(9) Some definitions of leadership come into what is termed *role theory* in sociology. This view sees the members of groups all interacting and playing their various roles with that of the leader being special. It depends on his ability to make clear the roles of everyone else within the group, and as such is the most indispensable role within the group. (10) Finally, leadership has been defined as the *initiation and maintenance* of group structure, whatever the leader does has more likelihood of structuring group behaviour than anything which other members of the group might do.

Overall, Stogdill feels that there is little unification in the various definitions outlined above. There do however seem to be some progressions over time. Increasingly, leadership has been viewed first as a matter of focusing group processes, then as the art of inducing compliance, and finally as a question of the differentiation of power and roles and the initiation of group structure. Whether or not leadership does in fact involve all this is still unresolved. Certainly they are not all necessary to theories of leadership. The main point is that a definition of leadership which might allow leaders to be easily picked out might still not say very much about what is involved in leadership.

Theories of Leadership

Just as with definitions, there have been a number of theories of leadership. Each has something in its favour and with the progression of time and expertise, they become better theories. Nevertheless, as will become clear, each also has its limitations. Basically, each theory of leadership has been concerned with attempting to explain both the nature of leadership and what is involved in it.

Great Man Theories

The early theories of leadership were based on the idea that leaders are born rather than made. They inherit certain qualities which ensure that they become leaders. If this were to be so, then the obvious question that has to be answered is: what are these qualities? Attempts to answer this question promoted the great man theories, by leading to the so-called *trait* theories of leadership.

There have been many studies carried out to explore the personality traits shared by great leaders, particularly if they come from families in which there is a history of leadership. Some traits do emerge fairly consistently, but these are all fairly obvious and mundane. For example: originality, popularity, sociability, judgement, aggression, humour, liveliness, amount of talking, intelligence (but not too much of it), hard work, expertise, degree of extraversion, and so on. However, the importance of any of these traits to leadership depends very much on the nature of the group which is being led and on what it is being led for. Also, it is worth mentioning that some characteristics are definitely *not* related to leadership: for example, age, height, weight, physique and appearance.

Environmental Theories

In reaction to the obvious genetic bias of the great man thoeries, there emerged some sheerly environmental theories of leadership. The import of these was that a leader emerges simply due to the exigencies of place, time and circumstances. Whether or not a person becomes a leader will then depend on the social needs and forces which exist at the time. Although it is no doubt true that crises produce leaders from people who would never otherwise have been so, one also needs to know how many crises do *not* do this; information which it is impossible to obtain. One also needs to know how many leaders emerge in non-crisis conditions, and also something about the qualities, if any, shared by those people to whom leadership is ascribed.

Genetic-environmental Theories

Inevitably, as a reaction against the purely genetic and purely environmental theories of leadership, theories were developed as a compromise between the two. These argued that leaders are people who inherit certain appropriate traits which are then realised only in specific societal and environmental conditions. People like Churchill and Hitler might be quoted as examples of this.

Theories of this sort were important in suggesting that attention be paid to the traits and motives of the leader, the images that people have of him and their motives in following him, the characteristics of the role he plays, and the institutional context in which it occurs. In this way leadership is seen as a relationship between people and not simply as a matter of personal characteristics or particular circumstances. Such a theory of leadership emphasises the interaction between whatever goals a leader might have and the goals of his followers.

Humanistic Theories

Following the humanistic reaction against behaviourism in many aspects of psychology, there have emerged humanistic theories of leadership. These stress the function of leadership as that of modifying the organisation of their groups in order to allow group members individual freedom

of action so that they can realise their own potentials and make a contribution to group goals. Sometimes such theories see effective leadership as that which allows followers to be maximally creative and self-
fulfilled. Doubtless, some leaders and some groups function like this,
but as a general theory of leadership it is too restricted, too narrow, and
perhaps amounts more to a prescription for one type of ideal leadership
than reflecting what actually happens.

Exchange Theories

An important theoretical standpoint in social psychology is that which
views all social interaction as an exchange. Any contribution to interaction is made at some personal cost but returns are received at cost to
those who give them. General social exchange is seen as continuing
because it is mutually rewarding.

In this context a leader makes unique contributions to the attain-
ments and goals of the group at some personal cost. But in return he
receives rewards of status and esteem from the group members. His role
as a leader will break down if he does not get enough in return for what
he puts in or if his own contributions are not judged to be of
sufficient value to merit the rewards he is receiving or to justify the
status and esteem he is given.

Interaction Theories

Nowadays, interaction theories of leadership are probably considered
the most important. Three types of these will be briefly described.
Homans suggests that the main role of a leader is to promote action,
interaction and sentiment amongst the group. The higher his rank then
the more his behaviour conforms to the norms of the group, the wider
are his interactions and the greater number of members for whom he
originates interaction.

Stogdill himself has a similar theory in which he suggests that group
members act in various roles and therefore reinforce the expectations of
all members that they will act in the same roles in the future. Any
potential for leadership is then seen as the degree to which the individual initiates and maintains group structure in interactions and does the
same for the expectations of the group members about what each other
will do.

Finally there is Fiedler's contingency theory of leadership which is
presently the most widely held. He divides leadership into two kinds:
that which is task or work oriented and that which is socially or
emotionally oriented. In general, the task oriented leader is the more

effective in both very easy and very difficult situations. The socially oriented leader is more effective in intermediate situations.

There is a great deal of research which shows that both types of leader emerge in many different groups. Often the task leader is the most influential and the social leader is the best liked. Frequently it is useful for a group to have both types, the task leader to see that the group aims are achieved and the social leader to provide some relief from sheer work. Occasionally in real-life situations the same man can fulfil both roles, especially when his position as leader has been ascribed to him and yet it is seen as deserved by his group members. Either type of leadership falls down if the leader spends too much time considering his own position, be this to be respected or to be liked. These two types of leadership will be returned to later.

Types and Functions of Leaders

A great deal of early research and theoretical effort was put into making analytic lists of the various functions that leaders fulfil. There are two kinds of such lists: those that stress types of leader and those that stress the functions a leader might have. A few representative examples of each will be discussed.

Types

Discussion of types of leader begins with Plato who felt that there were basically three types: a philosopher-statesman, a military commander, and a business man. More recently the following typologies have been suggested: charismatic, organisational, intellectual and informal. Or: persistent on-the-spot problem solvers, salient individuals with powerful influence, those nominated by their peers and therefore reasonably popular, and those who are simply elected.

Whatever breakdown is followed there are six major types which tend to recur
(1) authoritarian − a dominator
(2) democratic − a group developer
(3) executive − an administrator
(4) persuasive − a crowd rouser
(5) intellectual − an eminent man
(6) representative − a spokesman.

Of these, current research centres very much on the first two, the authoritarian and the democrat, which in fact amount to the task-oriented and social-emotionally oriented types mentioned earlier.

Functions

There have been many classifications of leaders according to their functions, the earlier text-books on social psychology always containing long lists of such functions. These were devised on the basis of observing leadership in everyday life. Without going into too much detail such lists would see leaders as: executives, planners, policy-makers, experts representative of the group, controllers of the group, rewarders and punishers, arbitrators and mediators, exemplars, symbols, scapegoats, surrogates for individual responsibility, ideologists, father figures, and so on.

Laboratory research into the functioning of small groups produced slightly different sets of functions. One breakdown for example is into a leader: maintaining standards of performance, giving nurture, and acting according to the immediate task at hand. Such an analysis and others like it again amount to redescriptions of task and social-emotional leaders, or leadership functions.

It is very doubtful that either structural or functional typologies of leadership can ever manage to list all the possible acts that a leader might make. So much will depend on the man, the circumstances in which the group forms and meets, the nature of the group itself, the task they face, and so on. In this sense each situation is unique. Also, to list all the functions and types of leadership is simply descriptive; it provides nothing in the way of explanation for what is going on. Both theoretically and practically it is important to know how to train leaders or how to provide the appropriate conditions in which they can emerge.

Identifying Leaders

Although it was shown above that some sort of interactional theory of leadership is likely to be appropriate, there are some studies which show that leaders can sometimes be identified on the basis of three types of characteristic: their skills, relationships with the group and some items which are purely personal.

Important *skills* include: social-interpersonal, technical, administrative, intellectual, achievement, friendliness, supportiveness in the task, and motivation. *Relationships* with members of the group include concern for welfare and concern that the group coheres. Personal items include such qualities as being well balanced, cultured or even attractive.

If these factors are important in identifying leaders, it must mean that not everyone within a group has the same potential for leadership. Although it is conceivable that virtually anybody could become a leader in some situation if he is given enough training, this will not normally happen. People differ markedly with respect to the characteristics mentioned above. The important question then becomes, when leaders are not ascribed to their position, how do they actually emerge?

Emergent Leadership

This is possibly the most important topic in leadership research and theory and a great deal has been written about it. The main factors which govern the emergence of leaders are: personal, group and peripheral. These will be dealt with in turn.

Personal Factors

(1) Talking. The member of a group who talks more and generally participates more in the group is likely to emerge as a leader. This does not simply relate to sheer amount of participation and talking, since most groups develop standards of quality as well. However, the person who makes an important point near the beginning or end of a discussion is more likely to emerge as a leader than he who makes a point in the middle. Leaders also tend to recover from interruption faster than non-leaders.

(2) Interaction. People differ with respect to how well they can initiate and maintain interaction, and how well they can do so in various situations (small as against large groups for example). Clearly, the person who is good at this — often called *expansiveness* — is likely to emerge as a leader.

(3) Miscellaneous. There are a number of factors based on personality or behaviour which do not fit into any obvious category and yet which have been shown to be related to emergent leadership. For example, leaders are more likely to emerge in people who initiate new and spontaneous contributions to the group, who allow the group to be relatively free rather than constricted, and who tend to relinquish their authority at appropriate moments. These three factors are important even in relatively authoritarian groups.

Group Factors

In general, leadership tends to transfer from one group to the next. All other things being equal, a leader who emerges in one group is likely to emerge again in another, particularly if the tasks involved are similar and if the other members of the groups tend to have similar roles and functions. However, there are a number of characteristics of groups which influence this transfer of emergent leadership.

(1) Task. It is obvious that different tasks demand different skills. Such skills may be distinguished along task or socio-emotional lines or with respect to intellectual or physical prowess. A person who emerges as the captain of a football team will not necessarily have the right characteristics to lead a group of school-teachers. A person who can lead a task force on the streets of Belfast will not necessarily be able to organise a field hospital. However, the person who is able to combine the task oriented and socio-emotionally oriented approaches to leadership is the one who will have the most carry over from one group to another.

(2) Variations in groups. To some extent emergent leadership depends on the number of leadership attempts which are made within the group. Attempts to assume leadership are more frequent in groups in which: (a) there are differences in social status (b) the group members are highly motivated, and (c) the task is difficult rather than easy. There also tend to be more attempts when the rewards for leadership are high.

Research in this area shows that leaders do not tend to emerge due to chance factors or some sort of discrimination, but through an interaction between various attempts which are made to assume leadership and the judgements which are made of these by the members of the group. One fairly comprehensive study concluded that there are six factors which are particularly facilitative of attempts to assume leadership: (a) larger rewards, (b) the likelihood of success of the task, (c) the general acceptance of the attempts, (d) tasks which require much decision on the part of the group, (e) having more information than the other members of the group, and (f) having a status recognised by the group members acquired from some previous experiences.

(3) Size. As might be expected there tends to be an inverse relationship between group size and possibilities for leadership. The larger the group the less likely it is for an individual to emerge as a leader. Also, the quality of leadership tends to change with the size of the group. The larger the group then the more demands are made on the leader and the more authoritarian he tends to become and tends to be expected to become. As this happens there is an attendant decrease in efficiency.

(4) Structure. Stogdill describes groups as going through four phases in

their development: (a) *forming* (coming together), (b) *storming* (struggles for power and position), (c) *norming* (developing norms), and (d) *performing* (solving the task or problem). Groups will only function well if these stages allow the differentiation of roles to occur, arguably the most important of which is the leadership role. This is likely to emerge in the storming stage.

Peripheral Factors

(1) The different forms of *communication* network can not only affect the functioning of a group but can also have a direct impact upon leadership and its emergence. This was demonstrated very clearly in an important study carried out by Leavitt (1951). He set up a series of five person groups each of which had a problem to solve. The members of each of these groups were given some of the information relevant to the solution of the problem, but they could only communicate this to one another according to predetermined channels which Leavitt set up. The four patterns he constructed are shown in Figure 16.1 with the circles representing group members and the lines possible avenues of communication.

Figure 16.1: Patterns of Communication from Leavitt's Study

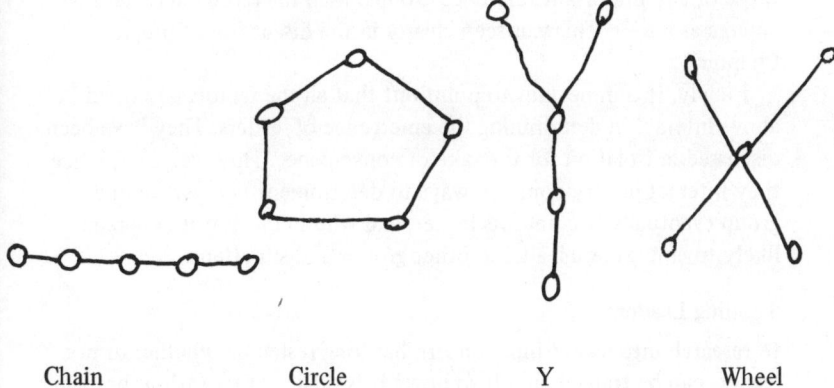

Chain   Circle   Y   Wheel

In describing the results of this study it is simpler to speak merely of the extremes – the circle and the wheel – since these represent the main findings, the results from the other types of structure endorsing the general findings by occupying intermediate positions. In the circle each member of the group can communicate with two others. There is equality but no opportunity for the emergence of leadership; there is no centrality to the group. Such groups solved the problems less efficiently and in longer times than for example the wheel formations, but the group members *on average* felt that they had enjoyed being group members rather more than did the wheel members, on average.

By contrast, the wheel has one person who is in a central position in the communication network. He can communicate with all other group members who in turn can communicate with him, even though they cannot communicate with one another. This was the most efficient group at problem solving, although it was only the obvious leader of the group who particularly enjoyed the experience.

(2) Personal Space. As mentioned in Chapter 12, leaders tend to gravitate to the head of a table, a position which in itself tends to facilitate leadership. Personal space is used to demonstrate physically the various roles that might exist in a group. So a leader tends to have a greater area of space around him than his followers.

(3) Norms. Norms external to the group and other groups to which they can refer often act as regulators of group behaviour and hence help to determine emergent leadership. The more a particular member of the group happens to internalise and then express the group norms and those of any important reference groups, then the more likely he is to emerge as leader. This was seen clearly in the discussion of prejudice in Chapter 15.

Finally, it is important to point out that all the factors described above interact in determining the emergence of leaders. They have been discussed in isolation for the sake of convenience. However, in practice they interact in very complex ways to determine which person in a group eventually becomes its leader, and whether or not that person is likely to emerge as a leader in other groups and situations.

Training Leaders

In research into leadership. concern has long rested on whether or not leaders can be trained, and if so how? It is obvious that various branches of society believe that they can since they have set up complex programmes for so doing (the armed services perhaps provide the best example, although there are many examples from civilian life as well). Some early research, mainly with school children showed that the members of groups do seem to benefit from training in leadership. Although the actual techniques used are rarely described in any detail, they can be roughly categorised into three types.

(1) Informational. This is traditional scholastic training in the form of lectures describing how leaders behave. Although there seem to be some gains in performance through this, it is clear that the information passes only in one direction and the situation is very inflexible. Those who are known already to have a reasonable potential for leadership seem to gain most from this type of training.

(2) Experiential. Experiential training in leadership takes the form either of role-playing or sensitivity training in T group situations as described in Chapter 14. Role playing does not seem to promote effective leadership and sensitivity training seems to promote only democratic styles of leadership, at least insofar as the individuals learn to share responsibility. Productivity goes down however.

(3) Combined. Mainly in which lectures are combined with sensitivity training. Although this sounds a reasonable idea it has not been thoroughly tested in its effectiveness in training leaders.

Group Effectiveness

A final discussion point in this chapter concerns the way in which various types or styles of leader lead to varying effectiveness in their groups. The impetus for this research area came from what is now regarded as a classic study by Lewin, Lippett and White (1939). Using boys staying in camps and giving them various normal camp problems to solve, they set up three styles of leadership and watched their development over the course of time. The three styles were:
(a) authoritarian — all decisions made by the leader,
(b) democratic — in which the leader is active, friendly and promotes participation in group decisions by the group members,
(c) laissez-faire — where the leader is friendly but completely passive.

In general, the findings were that the democratic style of leadership was most effective under almost all conditions, certainly producing very high cohesion in its groups. The authoritarian style was even more effective than this, *when the leader was present.* However, if he was absent for any reason, the group members did very little. The laissez-faire style was equally inefficient under all conditions. One aspect of group effectiveness which both this study and that of Leavitt, described above, does highlight, is that care needs to be taken in deciding exactly what is meant by this. It does not just mean how efficiently the group can solve problems or carry out tasks; it also means how content the members of the group are at being in the group. In the long term, a highly efficient group with disgruntled members may well break up.

Results such as these have clear bearing on Fiedler's contingency theory of leadership. A search was made for factors which are important to the relative effectiveness of task-centred versus socio-emotionally centred leadership. Fiedler proposed that there are three main factors involved:

(a) the leader's relationships with the other members of the group,
(b) the structure of the task to be done (whether it is hard or easy),
(c) whether or not the leader has *legitimate* authority.

Overall, as mentioned earlier, the authoritarian or task centred leader functions best when the conditions are easy or hard, and the democratic or socio-emotionally oriented functions best in the intermediate range.

The reasons for these differences are thought to be as follows. When a task is difficult, the group members tend to be keen to get the job going and will overlook any personal problems; they take directives easily. When the circumstances are neither good nor poor, then interpersonal problems raise their heads and the group orients better to the leader who is concerned with such problems. When the task is easy and the conditions favourable the group oriented leader may have too much time to dwell on his own somewhat enviable position in the group and even end up by losing some goodwill and forgetting the task altogether.

Summary Points

(1) A group is two or more persons in a state of social interaction, and contains members with differentiated roles and statuses.
(2) A group can be primary (face-to-face) or secondary and will vary according to its formality, what brings it about, its power relationships, and its communication patterns.
(3) Leadership has been defined in many ways, such definitions centring on leaders as focuses of group processes, as those who are good at inducing compliance, and as those who can initiate and maintain group structure.
(4) Theories of leadership have stressed genetics, the environment and interaction between the two. The interactional theories are the more important nowadays, particularly that which divides leadership into task-oriented (authoritarian) and socio-emotionally oriented (demo-

cratic).

(5) Attempts to list the types and functions of leaders can also best be summarised as ultimately being concerned with the two types of leadership just mentioned.

(6) Leaders can be identified according to their specific skills, their relationships with group members and various personal factors.

(7) Emergent leadership depends on a complex interaction between various personal factors, group factors and a number of peripheral factors, probably the most important of which are the communication networks existing in the group.

(8) The training of leaders can be done in a traditional information-giving way or by using various experiential approaches. Either way effectiveness is not easy to assess.

(9) Group effectiveness varies very much according to the type of leadership, particularly with respect to task-oriented and socio-emotionally oriented leadership.

Study Questions – 16

(1) Describe the different types of social groups that are found in hospitals. What sorts of leadership do these groups have?

(2) Have you observed any social situations in your training and your professional work in which leaders have emerged? What caused those particular persons to emerge?

(3) There are obvious moments in your professional life when you have to assume the role of a leader. Are you equal to such necessities? How could you learn to cope with more effectively? Could anybody be trained to such leadership?

(4) Try to draw up a full description of the communication networks that exist in a hospital in which you have worked. How much difference do you think that these networks make to group functioning and to the emergence of leaders?

(5) From your observations of patients and colleagues, do you think that there are some of them who would *never* emerge as leaders? If so, what are the characteristics of these people?

(6) What are the particular problems of leadership presented by your own working environment? How might these best be solved?

(7) How would you attempt to lead (persuade, direct, control, etc.) a patient or a colleague who is, (a) much older than yourself, (b) of a much higher social status, and (c) an important leader in his own right? What difficulties might such patients and colleagues present?

(8) Describe some hospital situations in which task-oriented leadership would be preferable to socio-emotional leadership and others in which the reverse might be true.

(9) To what extent do you think that leadership is affected by its social trappings such as uniforms, insignia, and badges of rank? What are the pros and cons of the various uniforms of the medical and paramedical professions?

(10) Consider the various difficulties and functions of leadership outlined in this chapter. Which of them apply particularly to your professional role? Why do the others not apply? Do different leadership functions apply to members of the different paramedical professions?

REFERENCES

Adorno, T.W. Frenkel-Brunswick, E. Levison, D.J. & Sanford, R.N. (1950), *The Authoritarian Personality*, NY: Harper & Row

Allport, G.W. (1961), *Pattern and Growth in Personality*, NY: Holt, Rinehart & Winston

Ames, A. Jr (1951) 'Visual Perception and the Rotating Trapezoidal Window', *Psychological Monographs*, vol. 65, no. 324

Argyle, M. (1964), *Psychology and Social Problems*, London: Methuen

Argyle, M. (1969), *Social Interaction*, London: Methuen

Arnold, M.B. (1960), *Emotion and Personality* (2 vols), NY: Columbia UP

Aronson, A. (1976), *The Social Animal* (2nd ed.) San Francisco: Freeman

Asch, S.E. (1946), 'Forming Impressions of Personality', *Journal of Abnormal and Social Psychology*, vol. 41, pp. 258-90

Asch, S.E. (1951), 'Effects of Group Pressure upon the Modification and Distortion of Judgement', in G. Guetzkow (ed.), *Groups, Leadership and Men*, Pittsburgh: Carnegie Press

Atkinson, J.M. (ed.) (1958), *Motives in Fantasy, Action and Society*, Princeton: Van Nostrand

Ayllon, J. (1963), 'Intensive Treatment of Psychotic Behaviour by Stimulus Satiation and Food Reinforcement', *Behaviour Research and Therapy*, vol. 1, pp. 53-62

Azrin, N.H. & Holz, W.C. (1966), 'Punishment', in W.K. Honig (ed.) *Operant Behaviour*, NY: Appleton-Century-Crofts

Bachrach, A.J.,Erwin, W.J. & Mohr, J.P. (1965), 'The Control of Eating Behaviour in an Anorexic by Operant Conditioning Techniques', in E.P. Ullman and L. Krasner (eds) *Case Studies in Behaviour Modification*, NY: Holt, Rinehart & Winston

Bandura, A. (1969), *Principles of Behaviour Modification*, NY: Holt, Rinehart & Winston

Bandura, A. & Walters, R.H. (1963), *Social Learning and Personality Development*, NY: Holt, Rinehart & Winston

Berscheid, E. & Walster, E.H. (1969), *Interpersonal Attraction*, Reading, Mass: Addison-Wesley

Bodmer, W.F. & Cavalli-Sforza, L.L. (1970), 'Intelligence and Race', *Scientific American*, October

Broadbent, D.E. (1958), *Perception and Communication,* London: Pergamon

Brown, R. (1966), *Social Psychology,* NY: Free Press

Bruner, J.S. & Goodman, C.C. (1947), 'Value and Need as Organising Factors in Perception', *Journal of Abnormal and Social Psychology* vol. 13, pp. 33-44

Bruner, J.S., Goodnow, J.J. & Austin, G.A. (1956), *A Study of Thinking,* NY: Wiley

Burt, C.L. (1961), 'Intelligence and Social Mobility', *British Journal of Statistical Psychology,* vol. 14, pp. 3-24

Byrne, D. & Nelson, D. (1965), 'Attraction as a Linear Function of Proportion of Positive Reinforcements', *Journal of Personality and Social Psychology,* vol. 1, pp. 659-63

Cannon, W.B. (1939), *The Wisdom of the Body* (2nd ed.) NY: Norton

Cattell, R.B. (1965), *The Scientific Analysis of Personality,* Harmondsworth: Penguin

Cautella, J.R. (1966), 'Treatment of Compulsive Behaviour by Covert Sensitisation', *Psychological Record,* vol. 16, pp. 33-41

Church, R.M. (1963), 'The Varied Effects of Punishment on Behaviour', *Psychological Review,* vol. 70, pp. 369-402

Cofer, C.N. & Appley, M.H. (1964), *Motivation: Theory and Research,* NY: Wiley

Darley, J. & Latane, B. (1968), 'Bystander Intervention in Emergencies: Diffusion of Responsibility', *Journal of Personality and Social Psychology*, vol. 8, pp. 377-83

Davis, C.M. (1928), 'Self-selection of diet by newly weaned children', *American Journal of Diseases of Children,* vol. 36, pp. 651-79

De Soto, C.B. (1960), 'Learning a Social Structure', *Journal of Abnormal and Social Psychology,* vol. 60, pp. 417-21

Dollard, J.C. & Miller, N.E. (1950), *Personality and Psychotherapy,* NY: McGraw-Hill

Ebbinghaus, H. (1913), *Memory,* (Trans. H.A. Roger and C.E. Bussenius) NY: Columbia University Press

Ekman, P. & Friesen, W.V. (1969), 'Nonverbal Leakage and Clues to Deception', *Psychiatry,* vol. 32, pp. 88-106

Epstein, S. (1967), 'Toward a Unified Theory of Anxiety', *Progress of experimental research in personality,* 4, 1-89, NY: Academic Press

Eriksen, B.A. & Eriksen, C.W. (1972), *Perception and Personality,* Morristown, NJ: General Learning Press

Erikson, E.H. (1963), *Childhood and Society* (2nd ed.) NY: Norton

Eysenck, H.J. (1953), *The Structure of Human Personality,* NY: Wiley

Eysenck, H.J. (1976), *Psychoticism as a Dimension of Personality,*
London: Hodder & Stoughton

Ferster, C.B. & Skinner, B.F. (1957), *Schedules of Reinforcement,*
NY: Appleton-Century-Crofts

Festinger, L. (1957), *A Theory of Cognitive Dissonance,* Evanston,
Ill: Row Peterson

Fincher, J. (1973), 'The Terman Study is 50 Years Old: Happy
Anniversary and Pass the Ammunition', *Human Behaviour,* vol. 2,
pp. 8-15

Freud, S. (1946), J. Strachey (ed.), *Standard Edition of Complete
Psychological Works of S. Freud,* London: Hogarth Press

Frijda, N.H. (1969), 'Recognition of Emotion', in L. Berkowitz
(ed.) *Advances in Experimental Social Psychology,* vol. 4, pp. 167-223

Getzels, J.W. & Jackson, P.W. (1962), *Creativity and Intelligence:
Explorations with Gifted Children,* NY: Wiley

Gewirtz, J.L. (1969), 'Mechanisms of Social Learning', in D.A. Geslin
(ed.) *Handbook of socialisation theory and research,* Chicago: Rand,
McNally

Goldiamond, L. (1965), 'Self Control Procedures in Personal Behaviour
Problems', *Psychological Reports,* vol. 17, pp. 851-68

Goldman, R., Jaffa, M. & Schachter, S. (1968), 'Yom Kippur, Air France,
Dormitory Food, and the Eating Behaviour of Obese and Normal
Persons', *Journal of Personality and Social Psychology,* vol. 10,
pp. 117-23

Gough, H.G. (1964), 'Identifying the Creative Person', Address to the
American Society of Value Engineers, Los Angeles

Guilford, J.P. (1967), *The Nature of Human Intelligence,* NY: McGraw-
Hill

Hall, C.S. (1951), 'The Genetics of Behaviour', in S.S. Steveson (ed.)
Handbook of Experimental Psychology, NY: Wiley

Hall, C.S. & Lindzey, G. (1970), *Theories of Personality* (2nd ed.) NY:
Wiley

Hall, E.T. (1959), *The Silent Language,* NY: Fawcett

Hall, R.V., Lund, D. & Jackson, D. (1968), 'Effects of Teacher Attention
on Study Behaviour', *Journal of Applied Behaviour Analysis,* vol. 1,
pp. 1-22

Hebb, D.O. (1949), *Organisation of Behaviour,* NY: Wiley

Heckhausen, H. (1967), *The Anatomy of Achievement Motivation,*
NY: Academic Press

Hess, E. (1965), 'Attitude and Pupil Size', *Scientific American,* vol. 212,
pp. 46-54

Homans, G. (1961), *Social Behaviour: Its Elementary Forms*, NY: Harcourt, Brace & World

Hubel, D.H. & Wiesel, T.N. (1965), 'Receptive Fields and Functional Architecture in 2 Nonstriate Visual Areas (18 and 19) of the Cat', *Journal of Neurophysiology*, vol. 28, pp. 229-89

Hull, C.L. (1943), *Principles of Behaviour*, NY: Appleton-Century-Crofts

Hunt, M. (1974), *Sexual Behaviour in the 1970s*, Chicago: Playboy Press

Isaacs, W., Thomas, J. & Goldiamond, I. (1960), 'Applications of Operant Conditioning to Reinstate Verbal Behaviour in Psychotics', *Journal of Speech and Hearing Disorders*, vol. 25, pp. 8-12

Izard, C.E. (1972), *The Face of Emotion*, NY: Appleton-Century-Crofts

Jacobson, E. (1964), *Anxiety and Tension Control*, Philadelphia: Lippincott

James, W. (1884), 'What is an Emotion?' *Mind*, vol. 9 pp. 188-205

Jensen, A.R. (1969), 'How Much Can We Boost IQ and Scholastic Achievement?' *Harvard Educational Review*, vol. 39, pp. 1-123

Jourard, S.M. (1966), 'An Exploratory Study of Body Accessibility', *British Journal of Social and Clinical Psychology*, vol. 5, pp. 221-31

Kaats, G.R. & Davis, K.E. (1972), 'The Social Psychology of Sexual Behaviour', in L.S. Wrightsman et al (eds), *Social Psychology in the Seventies,* Monterey: Wadsworth, Brooks/Cole

Kelly, G.A. (1955), *The Psychology of Personal Constructs*, NY: Norton

Kohler, W. (1925), *The Mentality of Apes*, NY: Harcourt Brace

Lazarus, R.S. (1968), 'Emotions and Adaptation: Conceptual and Empirical Relations', in W.J. Arnold (ed.), *Nebraska Symposium on Motivation*, Univ. of Nebr. Press, 193-8

Leavitt, H.J. (1951), 'Some Effects of Certain Communication Patterns on Group Performance', *Journal of Abnormal and Social Psychology*, vol. 46, pp. 38-50

Lettvin, J.Y.,Maturana, H.R., McCulloch, W.S. & Pitts, W.H. (1959), 'What the Frog's Eye Tells the Frog's Brain', *Proceedings of the I.R.E.*, vol. 47, pp. 1940-51

Lewin, K. Lippett, R. & White, R.K. (1939), 'Patterns of Aggressive Behaviour in Experimentally Created Social Climates', *Journal of Social Psychology*, vol. 10, pp. 271-99

Lindsay, P.H. & Norman, D.A. (1972), *Human Information Processing: An Introduction to Psychology*, NY: Academic Press

Lorenz, K. (1966), *On Aggression*, NY: Harcourt Brace

Luchins, A.S. (1957), 'Primacy-recency in Impression Formation', in

C.I. Harland et al, *The Order of Presentation in Persuasion*, NY: Yale U P

Maslow, A.H. (1954), *Motivation and Personality*, NY: Harper & Row

Maslow, A.H. (1972), *The Farther Reaches of Human Nature*, Harmondsworth: Penguin

Masters, W.H. & Johnson, V.E. (1966), *Human Sexual Responses*, Boston: Little, Brown

McClelland, C. (1961), *The Achieving Society*, Princeton: Van Nostrand

McDougall, W. (1908), *An Introduction to Social Psychology*, London: Methuen

McGeoch, J.A. & Iron, A.L. (1952), *The Psychology of Human Learning*(2nd ed.), NY: Longmans, Green

McGinnies, E. (1949), 'Emotionality and Perceptual Defence', *Psychological Review*, vol. 56, pp. 244-51

McGregor, D. (1960), *The Human Side of Enterprise*, NY: McGraw-Hill

Milgram, S. (1974), *Obedience to Authority*, NY: Harper & Row

Millenson, J.R. (1967), *Principles of Behaviour Analysis*, NY: Collier Macmillan

Miller, N.E. & Dollard, J. (1941), *Social Learning and Imitation*, New Haven: Yale U P

Neisser, U. (1964), 'Visual Search', *Scientific American*, vol. 210, pp. 194-210

Neisser, U. (1967), *Cognitive Psychology*, NY: Appleton-Century-Crofts

Pavlov, I.P. (1927), *Conditional Reflexes*, transl. G.V. Anrep, London: OUP

Peterson, L.R. & Peterson, M.J. (1959), 'Short-term Retention of Individual Verbal Items', *Journal of Experimental Psychology*, vol. 58, pp. 193-98

Postman, L.,Bruner, J. & McGinnies, E. (1948), 'Personal Values as Selective Factors in Perception', *Journal of Abnormal and Social Psychology*, vol. 43, pp. 143-54

Rogers, C.R. (1961), *On becoming a Person*, Boston: Houghton Mifflin

Sandford, R.N. (1936), 'The Effects of Abstinence From Food upon Imaginal Processes: A Preliminary Experiment', *Journal of Psychology*, vol. 2, pp. 129-36

Schachter, S. (1971), *Emotion, Obesity and Crime*, NY: Academic Press

Schachter, S. & Gross, L.P. (1968), 'Manipulated Time and Eating Behaviour', *Journal of Personality and Social Psychology*, vol. 10, pp. 98-106

Schachter, S. & Singer, J. (1962), 'Cognitive, Social, and Physiological of Emotional State', *Psychological Review*, vol. 69, pp. 373-99

Secord, P.F.S. & Backman, C.W.B. (1974), *Social Psychology* (2nd ed.),
    NY: McGraw-Hill
Sheldon, W.H. (1943), *Varieties of Temperament*, NY: Harper & Row
Sheldon, W.H. (1954), *Atlas of Man*, NY: Harper & Row
Skinner, B.F. (1938), *The Behaviour of Organisms*, NY: Appleton-
    Century
Spearman, C. (1927), *The Abilities of Man*, NY: Macmillan
Sperling, G. (1960), 'The Information Available in Brief Visual Present-
    ations', *Psychological Monographs*, vol. 74, no. 11
Spielberger, C.D. (ed.), (1966), *Anxiety and Behaviour*, NY: Academic
    Press
Stogdill, P.M. (1974), *Handbook of Leadership*, NY: Free Press
Strongman, K.T. (1978), *The Psychology of Emotion* (2nd ed.), NY & `
    London: Wiley
Terman, L.M. (1954), 'Scientists and Non-Scientists in a Group of 800
    Gifted Men', *Psychological Monographs*, vol. 68, no. 7
Thurstone, L.L. (1938), *Primary Mental Abilities*, Chicago: Univ. of
    Chic. Pr.
Torrance, E.P. (1962), *Guiding Creative Talent*, NJ: Prentice Hall
Voeks, V. (1964), *On Becoming an Educated Person: An Orientation
    to College*, (2nd ed.), Philadelphia; Founders
Wallas, G. (1926), *The Art of Thought*, NY: Harcourt, Brace
Watson, J.B. & Raynor, R. (1920), 'Conditioned Emotional Reactions',
    Journal of Experimental Psychology, vol. 3, pp. 1-14
Whiting, J.W. & Child, I.L. (1953), *Child Training and Personality*, New
    Haven: Yale U P
Whorf, B.F. (1940) 'Science and Linguistics', *Technical Review*, vol. 44,
    pp. 229-48
Winch, R.F. (1958), *Mate Selection: A Study of Complementary Needs*,
    NY: Harper & Bros
Wispe, L.G. & Dramarean, N.C. (1953), 'Physiological Needs, Word
    Frequency and Visual Duration Thresholds', *Journal of Experimental
    Psychology*, vol. 46, pp. 25-31
Witkin, H.A. and others (1954), *Personality Through Perception: An
    Experimental and Clinical Study*, NY: Harper & Row
Wolf, S. & Wolff, H.G. (1947), *Human Gastric Function*, Oxford: OUP
Wolpe, J. (1958), *Psychotherapy by Reciprocal Inhibition*, Stanford:
    Stanford Univ. Press
Zeigarnick, B. (1927), Uber das Behalten von erledigten und
    unerledigten Handlungen, *Psychological Forschung*, vol. 9, pp. 1-85

INDEX

abnormal behaviour 10, 45-63
abnormal thought 126-7
accident 146, 173
accommodation 101
accuracy 222-3, 228
achievement 161-2, 164, 192
active filtering and processing 106
activity 154
acuity 100-1, 110
adolescence 174, 231
Adorno, T.W. 174-5
adrenaline 135-6
aggression 11-12, 144-8, 166, 173,
   175, 254, 255
Allport, G.W. 106
Ames, J.R. 104
amnesia 87
anal zone 169
analysis by synthesis 97-8
anger 19, 131, 132, 134, 136, 137,
   140, 145, 149, 217, 219
animal studies 132
anorexia 54-5
anxiety 27, 40, 48, 50, 58, 127,
   131, 137, 139, 140, 141-4, 150,
   166, 169, 170, 173, 178, 227,
   242, 251
aphagia 156
Appley, M.H. 157
appraisal 137-8
Argyle, M. 201-11, 230-45
Arnold, M.B. 134, 137
Aronson, E. 240, 251
arousal 135-7, 143, 217, 231
Asch, S.E. 110, 215
assertive responses 50
association value 68-9
Atkinson, J.M. 161
attitude 246-61
attitude change 250-52, 258-9, 260
attraction 223-8
audience 252
Austin, G.A. 116
authoritarian personality 174-5
autonomic nervous system 133-4
aversion 58
avoidance 38, 48
Ayllon, J. 53

Azrin, N.H. 40

Bachrach, A.J. 54
Backman, C.W.B. 224, 226, 232-5,
   253
balance theory 224-5
Bandura, A. 175
behaviourism 17-22, 178
behaviour modification (therapy)
   45-63
behaviour therapists 56-7
belief 246-7, 255
Berscheid, E. 224
bicycles 42
blame 21
blindness 221
blinking 11, 26
Bodmer, W.F. 191
body contact 202
body language 201-12, 220
body type 167-8
brightness 99, 110
Broadbent, D.E. 106
Brown, R. 195-201, 222
Bruner, J.S. 108, 116
Byrne, D. 225
bystanders 237

Cannon, W.B. 133, 150
case histories 12, 52-6
categorisation 116-17
catharsis 147
cats 98-9
Cattell, R.B. 177, 180
Cautela, J.R. 58
Cavalli-Sforza, L.L. 191
centrality 215
cerebrotonia 167-8, 179
Child, I.L. 174
chimpanzees 41
choice 154
Church, R.M. 40
classification of motives 163
Cofer, C.N. 157
cognition 10, 41, 107-8, 112-29,
   134-8, 149, 163, 246-7, 259
cohesion 235
colour vision 35, 102, 110

285

communication 195-212, 262, 264, 273-4, 276
compliance 265
concept formation 115-18
condescension 197
conditioning, classical (respondent) 24-44, 45-63, 138-41, 150
conditioning, higher-order 30, 35-6, 43
conditioning, instrumental (operant) 24-44, 45-63, 138-41, 231
cone cells 99
confabulation 84
conformity 236-7, 256
conscience 168
consciousness 20
consolidation theory 67, 88
constancies 105-6, 110
constitution 167-8, 179
context 218-20
contingency theory 268
control 13-16, 17, 76, 131
convergence 101
coping 138
costs 235
covert sensitisation 58
creativity 65, 119-21, 187-8
credibility 252
culture 174-5, 180, 221-2, 257-8
curiosity 65

dark adaptation 99
Darley, J. 237
Darwin, C. 153, 190
Davis, C.M. 156
Davis, K.E. 160
day-dreaming 112
decay of memory 87-8
deception 220-1
deference 197
definition 9-23, 33, 112, 145, 152, 166, 182-3, 193
delusions 119-20
depth perception 91, 101-2, 104, 110
De Soto, C.B. 200
determinism 16-22
development 10, 168-71, 184, 253
diets 157, 191
discrimination 29-30, 34-5, 43, 115, 252-9
disease 46
disruption 64-5
dissonance 226, 250-1, 260
distance 199, 202-3, 274

dogs 25-30
Dollard, J.C. 175, 242
dominance 162, 204, 206
double alternation 121
Dramarean, N.C. 108
drive 152, 242

Ebbinghaus, H. 68, 79, 85
ectomorphy 167-8, 179
ego 45, 168, 176, 180
eidetic imagery 91, 92
Ekman, P. 220
elation 140
Electra complex 170
electro-convulsive shock 89
emergent leadership 271-5
emotion 10, 27, 48, 131-51, 192, 203-4, 216-22, 246-7, 259, 272
emotion, theories 132-41
emotional behaviour 138-41, 150
emotional education 149-50
emotional expression 216-22, 228
endomorphy 167-8, 179
Epstein, S. 143
Eriksen, B.A. 108
Eriksen, C.W. 108
Erikson, E.H. 171
errors 84
Erwin, W.J. 54
escape 38
esteem 235
euphoria 136
everyday learning 238
exchange theory 226-8, 242-3, 268
expectation 42
experience 18-22, 116, 131, 137, 171-4
experimental neurosis 30
experimental variables 12-16, 22
experimentation 12-16, 22
exploration 160, 164
extinction 27-8, 33-4, 43, 45, 49, 51, 56
extraversion 126, 177-8, 180, 214
eye movements 204-5
Eysenck, H.J. 177-8

facial expression 131, 204-5
family 262-3
fantasy 118-19, 233
faulty reasoning 124-5
fear 135, 139, 218
feedback 69, 73, 74, 208, 241
feeling 130-51, 199-200, 241, 246
Festinger, L. 250

Fiedler, J. 268, 276
field dependence and independence 109
fighting services 258
figural organisation 103-4
Finchter, J. 187
first impressions 214-15
flexibility 123
forgetting 65, 76-93
formal learning 239
formality 197, 263-4, 276
forms of address 196-7
free-association 118
free-will 16-22
Freud, S. 17, 142, 146-53, 168-71, 178-80
friendship 227
Friesen, W.V. 220
Frijda, N.H. 216
frogs 98-9
frustration 147, 219, 254

gastric fistula 158
generalisation 28-9, 34-5, 43, 115, 116, 176
genetics 17
Gestalt laws 103-4, 110
gesture 203-4, 220
Getzels, J.W. 120
Gewirtz, J.L. 175
gifted children 186
Goldiamond, L. 52, 59
Goldman, R. 157
Goodman, C.C. 108
Goodnow, J.J. 116
Gough, H.G. 187
great man theories 266-7
Gross, L.P. 156
group effectiveness 275-6
groups 262-78
group size 272
group structure 272
Guilford, J.P. 183

habits 25, 41, 46
Hall, C.S. 178
Hall, E.T. 202
Hall, R.V. 64
happiness 132
Hebb, D.O. 182
Heckhausen, H. 161
heredity-environment 188-92, 267
Hess, E. 113
hoarding 53
Holz, W.C. 40

Homans, G. 235, 242
hormones 159
housing 259
Hubel, D.H. 98
Hull, C.L. 41
humanistic theories 267
hunger 154, 155-7, 164
Hunt, M. 159
hyperphagia 156
hypothalamus 134, 156, 157

icon 81
id 168, 180
identity 232
illusions 95-6, 110
impressions of personality 213-29
influence 265
information processing 94-111
injections 26
insight 41
instinct 146, 154-5, 169
intelligence 182-97
intention 18-22, 146
interaction theory 268
interference theory 89-90, 92
interpersonal relationships 195-212
interruption 19, 87
interviewing 239
intimacy 197, 202
introversion 177-8, 180, 214
I.Q. 162, 182-97
Irion, A.L. 67
Isaacs, N. 52
Izard, C.E. 148, 149, 216

Jackson, D. 64
Jackson, P.W. 120
Jacobson, E. 50
Jaffa, M. 157
James, W. 133, 150
Jensen, A.R. 191
Johnson, V.E. 159
Jourard, S.M. 202
judgement 213-29

Kaatz, G.R. 160
Kelly, G.A. 173-4, 178, 180
kissing 202
Kohler, W. 41

laboratory studies 13-16, 22
language 10, 113-15
Latane, B. 237
latency 27, 33, 170
Lazarus, R.S. 137

leadership 257, 262-78
leadership, functions 270
leadership, identification 270
leadership, training 274-5
leadership, types 269-70
learning 9, 10, 15, 24-75, 230-45
learning curves 66, 74
Leavitt, H.J. 273
Lettvin, J.Y. 98
Lewin, K. 275
lie detectors 134
Likert scales 249
Lindsay, P.H. 97
Lindzey, G. 178
linguistic relativity 114-15
Lippett, R. 275
long-term memory 82-3, 92
Lorenz, K. 164
love 139, 223-8
Luchins, A.S. 214
Lund, D. 64

McClelland, C. 161
McDougall, W. 155
McGeoch, J.A. 67
McGinnies, E. 108
McGregor, D. 153
maladaptive behaviour 45-63
management of learning 64-75
Maslow, A.H. 163, 164, 172
Masters, W.H. 159
maturation 24
mazes 32
meaningfulness 68-9, 86
measurement 9-22, 27, 33, 131, 154,
    166, 176-8, 213, 249-50, 260
medical model 45-63
medical problems 45-63
memory 9, 10, 15, 65, 76-93
memory trace 87-8
menstruation 159
mental age 182
mental disorder 45-63
mental practice 80, 86
mental retardation 184-6
mesomorphy 167-8, 179
messages 151-2
Milgram, S. 136-7
Millenson, J.R. 140
Miller, N.E. 175, 242
mnemonics 83, 92
modelling 51
models of man 16-22
Mohr, J.P. 54
mongolism 185

mother and child 36, 162, 174-6
motivated forgetting 86-7
motivation 10, 15, 64, 65, 76, 86-7,
    92, 108, 152-65, 171-4, 209,
    235, 238, 272
motive 152, 175
movement 217-18
multiplexity 248
muscle activity 113, 115

nature/nurture 188-92, 267
need 152, 225
Neisser, U. 8, 97, 103, 106
Nelson, D. 225
neurosis 141-2
neuroticism 177-8, 180
neutral region 249
nonsense syllables 68-9, 92
Norman, D.A. 97

obedience 236-7
obesity (overeating) 53-4, 59, 60,
    136, 156
objectivity 12
observation 10-12, 22
occupation 186-7, 258
Oedipus complex 169-70
old age 184
operant behaviour 30-44
operant level 31-2
orgasm 159
overlap 101

pain 160, 164
paired associates 71, 77, 79, 92
parachutists 143
parallax 101
part versus whole learning 67
pattern recognition 94-9, 110
Pavlov, I.P. 25, 49
perception 94-111, 172, 207, 213-29,
    231, 238
perceptual selectivity 106
performance 66
personal characteristics 198-9
personality 10, 166-8, 213-29, 249,
    265, 271
perspective 101
persuasion 251-2, 260, 265
Peterson, L.R. 82
Peterson, M.J. 82
phenomenology 18-22, 171-4
phenylketonuria 185
philosophy 9
phobias 142

physiology 130-51
physique 166-7
Piaget, J. 79
pituitary 158
political attitudes 248
polygraph 134
Postman, L. 108
power 162, 253, 264
practice 66
predictability 18-21, 178
prejudice 252-61
primacy 214
primary groups 262-3
proactive interference 90-1
probability 27, 33
problem solving 114
programmed instruction 72-3
progressive narrowing 59
projection 222
psychoanalysis 118, 170, 175
psychometrics 176-8, 180
psychotherapy 57, 62, 159, 172
psychoticism 177
punishment 39-41, 43, 47, 175, 227

race 190-2
rage 139, 173
rapport 191, 209
rationality 18, 132, 137
rats 31-4
Raynor, R. 138
reality principle 168
reasoning 121-5
recall 77
recency 214
reciprocal inhibition 58
recognition 77-8
reflex 25, 168
reinforcement 26-44, 45-63, 65, 115,
   176, 178, 225, 226, 235
reinforcement, partial 37-8
reinforcement, schedules 37-8
reinforcement, secondary 36-7
relaxation 50
relearning 78
relief 140
reminiscence 79
response set 222-3
responsibility 21
retina 99
retrieval 84-5, 92
retroactive interference 89-90
rod cells 99
Rogers, C.R. 171-2, 178, 180
roles and role-learning 232-5, 239-40,

262, 276

salivation 25
Sandford, R.N. 157
sarcasm 19, 161
satiation 51-2, 54, 155
savings method 78
scapegoating 254
Schachter, S. 135-7, 150, 156-7
schizophrenia 52-4, 126
school performance 186
scientific method 9-23, 131
secondary groups 263
Secord, P.F.S. 224, 226, 232-5, 253
self 171-4, 176, 178, 180
self-actualisation 163, 173, 192
self-confidence 60, 121
self-control 57-60, 61
sensory information storage 80-1, 92
separation anxiety 144
serial anticipation 77
serial position effect 68, 92
sex 50, 60, 157, 158-60, 164,
   169-70, 175
shaping 32, 53
Sheldon, W.H. 167-8, 179
shock 39, 139, 236
short-term memory 81-2, 92
shuttle box 38
Singer, J. 135
skills 64-75, 86, 207-11
Skinner, B.F. 31, 49, 243
Skinner box 31-2, 64, 69, 139
smoking 251
snoring 49
social behaviour 10, 172, 174-6,
   195-278
social class 189-90
social isolation 48
social learning (socialisation) 147,
   174-6, 230-45, 270
social skills 207-11, 230-45, 270
social style 205-7
social symbols 200-1
social techniques 201-12
solidarity 195-201, 210
somatotonia 167-8, 179
Spearman, C. 183
speech 205
Sperling, G. 81-2, 103
Spielberger, C.D. 143
spontaneous recovery 28
sport 24, 71, 160
stabilised retinal image 103, 110
statistics 15-16, 22, 178

status 195-201, 210, 253, 255, 260, 263, 272, 276
stealing 53
stereotype 168, 223, 252
stimuli 25-44
Stogdill, P.M. 265, 266, 268, 273
storage tank 82-3
Strongman, K.T. 216
study habits 59, 69-70
study questions 22-3, 43-4, 62-3, 74-5, 92-3, 111, 128-9, 151, 164-5, 180-1, 193-4, 211-12, 228-9, 244-5, 260-1, 277-8
stuttering 48
sulking 59
superego 168, 180
systematic desensitisation 50-1, 58

talking 271
teaching 65
teaching machines 72-3
television 12
temper tantrums 56
template matching 95
Terman, L.M. 120, 187
thalamus 133, 134
thematic apperception test 161-2
thinking 65, 112-129
thirst 157-8, 164
Thomas, J. 52
thought strategies 117-18
Thurstone, L.L. 183
toilet training 169, 176
tolerance of ambiguity 121, 255
T (training) groups 240-2

traits 175-8, 266-7
transfer of training 70-2, 74
trustworthiness 252
twin studies 188-9

valence 247
verbalisers 83
virginity 159
viscerotonia 167-8, 179
visualisers 83
visual search 106-7
Voeks, V. 69
voluntary behaviour 30-44

Wallas, G. 119
Walster, E.H. 224
Walters, R.H. 175
Watson, J.B. 138
White, R.K. 275
Whiting, J.W.
Whorf, B.F. 114
Wiesel, T.N. 98
will-power 57, 171
Winch, R.F. 225
Wispe, L.G. 108
Witkin, H.A. 109
Wolf, S. 134
Wolff, H.G. 134
Wolpe, J. 50
work 153

Yom Kippur 157

Zeigarnik, B. 87